JOURNEY
TO A
MIRACLE

WHEN FAITH WAS THE ONLY CURE

JEFF SCISLOW

aBM

Published by:
A Book's Mind
PO Box 272847
Fort Collins, CO 80527
www.abooksmind.com

ISBN 978-1-939828-86-6

www.JourneyToAMiracle.com
Jeff@JourneyToAMiracle.com

Acclaim for Journey to a Miracle

I remember visiting Jeff in the hospital. I went to offer him some company, comfort, and encouragement. Instead, I was the one who left encouraged by him! Jeff's optimism was contagious; his faith never wavered—the outcome was a miraculous healing.

DAVID LINGER
EXEC. VP, REGIONAL DIRECTOR,
RE/MAX NORTH CENTRAL,INC.

I have followed Jeff's business success for years. Year after year, he performs at the top of his game. When faced with a life-threatening disease, he rose to the occasion and never gave up. His example of determination, perseverance, and unwavering faith in God is one we can all gainstrength from.

GARY KELLER
FOUNDER & CHAIRMAN,
KELLER WILLIAMS REALTY INTERNATIONAL

With such a powerful and compelling story set forth in this book, the greatest tragedy would be to read it and decide 'it could not happen to me' or someone you love. Jeff Scislow is a man who dares to believe in God's timeless truths and his life shines as a beacon. Take his story as proof that God can and will prove Himself strong to those who believe.

JANE PARK SMITH
MS. AMERICA 2008

Do miracles happen? Does God answer prayers? Can faith heal? My spiritual upbringing engrained a 'Yes' to all three questions. However, when faced with a life threatening illness, I witnessed Jeff Scislow, by what seemed like an iron will of faith, receive a personal 'Yes' to each of those questions.

I'd witnessed determination, focus, persistence, inquisitiveness, and a charming personality serve him well in his business, and then I admired his ability to apply those same qualities in his battle for life. His greatest partner, faith in the Almighty, coupled with those qualities that make Jeff Scislow what he is . . . allows us to enjoy him and his powerful spirit today.

HOWARD BRINTON
FOUNDER AND CEO, STAR POWER SYSTEMS

Journey to a Miracle is one of those books that gives a pure injection of love, hope, and faith. I truly believe that as some read this book, miracles of healing will take place. One thing for sure, all who read it will come away refreshed and in awe of the goodness of God.

PATRICIA KING
EXTREME PROPHETIC

This book is a 'profile in courage.' I was with Jeff when he received the diagnosis and can say without reservation that without his bold reaction, he would not be alive today. Many of my friends bailed on Jeff when he took this radical direction, but I stuck with him, even though it stretched my faith to places it had not been before. I have used his story countless times to encourage others to choose life in the face of devastating diagnoses.

DAVE HOUSHOLDER
PASTOR, ROBINWOODCHURCH.COM

While serving in the Marine Corps in the latter 1970s, Jeff consistently performed as one of the most outstanding Marines under my supervision. His determination and the 'fight' that he displayed at that time is evident throughout this book as he overcame obstacles, most importantly, the fight for his life.

SERGEANT MAJOR JOHN M. ROBERSON
USMC, RETIRED

I've personally known Jeff for many years. His drive and determination not only set him apart as a person but also made him one of the most successful sales associates within the worldwide RE/MAX organization. After receiving a medical 'death sentence,' Jeff rose to the occasion and met the challenge head on with a unique sense of optimism. As one of thousands who witnessed the events unfold during Jeff's period of illness, I can say without hesitation that his strong faith, fighting attitude, and expectation of a miracle are the reasons he is alive today.

Journey to a Miracle explores the depths of Jeff's experience, the choices he made, and the miracle he received. Prepare yourself for victory, as you allow this book to inspire and impact your life.

MARGARET KELLY
CEO, RE/MAX INTERNATIONAL

I believe the Lord initially led Jeff to the medical clinic where I practice and entrusted me to care for His servant. Despite the life threatening diagnosis and 'medicine's' inability to find a cure, Jeff was steadfast in his belief that the Lord would see him through. His faith in the Lord would be the 'shining star' leading him through his darkest hour. His is a story to inspire us all!

SCOTT PODRATZ, PA-C
FAMILY PRACTICE/URGENT CARE MEDICINE

When I arrived at the intensive care unit of the hospital I was warned to wash my hands and be careful around Jeff, as he could die from common germs. While with Jeff, the doctor came in with the test results. The doctor hesitated with the weight of the news he was about to deliver. In short the doctor told Jeff, 'You're the man who got hit by lightning'—as there was no reason 'why Jeff'—but the fact was Jeff received the deadly diagnosis.

What amazed me was Jeff's response! After being told he would die from the disease, Jeff somehow became excited by the details of the bad news as he sat up in bed, as weak as he was, got a sparkle in his eye, and said, 'Wow, won't this make a great testimony when God heals me!'

Jeff's unnatural response began this amazing journey of faith. Others would be overwhelmed by the report. Jeff was fascinated by every detail and became excited by the news. He believed and expected that the hand of God would perform a miracle in his life and began right then telling everyone about it!

As a minister that has had miracles in and around my life, I am deeply touched by the miraculous healing that Jeff is now testifying to. This is not just a book on a miracle happening to Jeff but a book that will open the door to a miracle happening in your life and in the life of those that you love!

DOUG STANTON
DOUG STANTON MINISTRIES INTERNATIONAL

Jeff's story provides tools available to each of us to create the life we desire, regardless of the challenges we face.

DAN PROESCHEL
D.D.S.

To see Jeff on the other side of his crisis gives me faith to believe that anything is possible! He shows by example that we can overcome insurmountable odds and find greater purpose in life.

ROB KETTERLING
LEAD PASTOR, RIVER VALLEY CHURCH

Jeff's journey has been one of faith, honor, and integrity. A must read story for those wanting to be truly inspired.

TOM ECKERT
INTERNATIONAL 747 CAPTAIN

Jeff Scislow's amazing and inspiring story confirms the Hashem (the Almighty in Hebrew) hears our faithful prayers and strengthens us as He did Jeff.

RUDY BOSCHWITZ
U.S. SENATOR

CONTENTS

INTRODUCTION

Take a moment and consider the following: When hit with a significant event that rocks your world, puts the pressure on, costs you dearly, or somehow interrupts your life in an unpleasant way, how do you personally respond? Are your responses deliberate or unpredictable? Do you take action, or do you feel helpless? What about your emotions . . . are they cool, calm, and collected or filled with stress and anxiety or perhaps even anger? How satisfied have you been with your method of response and the resulting outcomes?

Over the years, I've observed great contrast in the human response to the challenges we all encounter. As a result of these observations, as well as numerous personal experiences, I've become convinced that the outcome of any given challenge is significantly tied to the response given it. I've found that any response has a tendency to fall into one of two predominant and opposing categories: faith-based or fear-based. Consider the differences: Faith refreshes and promises to deliver, while fear grips and ultimately destroys.

When a person *chooses* to believe in a positive outcome through faith, it births hope. Hope in turn inspires and fuels the journey toward the goal of what is expected through faith. Outcomes of faith-based actions are overwhelmingly positive and at times even miraculous. Fear-based responses on the other hand, while they could motivate one into taking an initial action, oftentimes immobilize and keep a person from taking any action at all, leaving its victim in a realm of self-pity, depression, or worse.

So, why wouldn't everyone respond from a position of faith instead of fear when facing some of life's biggest hurdles or surprises? Perhaps some are not sure what they believe. Others may not know what to have faith in. Still, others may be unsure what faith is all about. In fact, the entire issue of *faith* can be confusing and difficult to wrap one's mind around.

There is much to learn about faith from the Old Testament account of Job. Job was a man of integrity, upright in all his ways. In fact, he was described as the most righteous man in all the land. In addition to being a man of great character, he was also a man of great wealth. His possessions were vast in number, which included land, animals, and servants. One day, in the midst of his great success, calamity struck with a vengeance. In a matter of hours, one catastrophe after another stripped him of everything he owned! Shortly thereafter, boil-like sores broke out all over his body. Next, his wife and friends turned on him and accused him falsely of things he must have done to bring such calamity upon himself. Even though Job was financially, physically, and emotionally devastated, he *chose* to respond out of faith and not out of fear in the midst of his dire circumstances.

As a result of Job's *faith* response to these challenges—a response he persisted in each and every day—he was later rewarded with the restoration of his health and the *doubling* of the great wealth he once had. What was this faith that Job had and where did he get it?

Job simply chose to believe in the promises of God that are recorded in the most published book in the history of the world—the Bible. No matter how devastating his circumstances, he made a conscious decision to believe in the promises rather than what he visually saw, emotionally felt, or had a tendency to otherwise believe.

Job's is not an isolated story of overcoming challenging circumstances through faith. *Today* there are incredible, even miraculous stories of faith taking place all around us. Through faith people are being delivered from financial woes, relational issues, unpleasant medical diagnoses, and the many crazy and sometimes bizarre situations we all face in life.

Faith has operated mightily in my life for years, and I've learned that three basic components must be at work in order for faith to produce the type of amazing outcomes of which it is capable. First, it is essential to identify a promise from the Bible that fits your situation. If you have need for healing, for example, then locating passages that promise healing from a sickness or disease is your initial step. Second, make a conscious choice to believe in the promise(s) no matter what you may be witnessing around you. Rest assured, doubt will creep in, but you must stand firm on what you believe. Do not waver or allow fear to derail your faithful expectation. Third, be patient and continually trust that the promise is for you and will come to pass in God's perfect timing, not necessarily yours.

While there are additional components of exercising your faith, such as discernment, wisdom, and common sense, the above three are foundational when putting your faith into action. Once you've made up your mind to engage your faith, a sense of peace and assurance will rise up within you. As you walk by faith and not by sight, you'll have placed yourself in the realm of unlimited possibility, even the miraculous.

The Bible defines faith as the evidence of things not seen, and the substance of things hoped for (see Hebrews 11:1). This means that you must believe that you have that which you seek before the evidence or substance has appeared. This must become a conviction because it is the key to unlocking the divine power of the promises. Then, out of this conviction, you must take action by living and speaking words that are consistent with the promises. After all, faith without action is useless.

IV

So, how can you understand these promises and obtain the faith necessary to overcome the challenges of life? Faith arrives then grows by reading and knowing about the promises (that too is a promise). While the promises are free and available to all, each of us is reminded that we must believe in order to receive the manifestation of the great promises found in the Bible. We're encouraged to follow by example: . . . *be an imitator of those who through faith and patience inherit the Promises* (Hebrews 6:12). These promises are available to you. They are available to all who seek, who ask, and who would knock to have the door of understanding opened, and through them nothing will be impossible for you. There is no mountain so high you cannot climb it, no valley so low you cannot travel its barren ground, and no ocean so deep you cannot navigate its rough waters.

As you'll learn in the pages ahead, I've had the privilege of walking through the valley of the shadow of death and have experienced the miraculous power as a result of faith in these promises. They can and will produce miracles in your life and are your unmatched weapons in overcoming fear and rising above any challenge you may be facing now or in the future. Allow this true story—which escalates in intensity and severity—to bless you, inspire you, and propel you into a new level of faith, possibility, and empowerment. Nothing is impossible to those who believe!

CHAPTER 1

— The Tsunami of Challenges Begins —

Consider it all joy when you encounter various trials, knowing that
the testing of your faith produces endurance.
—JAMES 1:2-3

Chapter 1

My plane landed safely under the overcast skies of Seattle in March 2000. I was filled with anticipation at seeing twenty very successful real estate associates from around the country. I knew about a dozen of them and was anxious to meet the others who had also been invited to this special gathering. Equally exciting was the fact that we had been hand-picked to review a new Internet technology and possibly to become involved with its anticipated success. My personal invitation to attend this gathering was not only exciting but an honor. I was part of a tremendous group.

Our first day at the corporate facility was eventful. We met the president and officers of the company and visited with the heads of the technology, accounting, and personnel departments. We had the opportunity to tour the entire facility and visit with many of the fifty employees who had developed the new Internet product, which would provide online service to real estate agents around the country.

This was the ultimate dot-com company for the industry that I had come to love. And there I was, right in the midst of this incredible opportunity. Over the next few days, our group was offered the opportunity to become members of the company's advisory panel. If we agreed to accept the proposal and responsibilities that came with it, we would receive stock options and other perks such as the opportunity to buy company stock at pre-offering prices.

We saw the vision, and it was awesome. We understood the need in the real estate industry, recognized how this new product could fill that need, and saw the strategic plan of how the company would grow as a result. The company and its employees had listened to our ideas and welcomed them; they realized the need for our professional input and business acumen, and we began to feel like a family within just a few days. The company had just signed a major training contract with the National Association of Realtors, a contract that would provide national exposure to over 700,000 Realtors and pave the way for the company to roll out its new products and services. The timing, the people, the product, and the need could not have been better. In addition, the Internet product was not limited only to real estate professionals; it was an awesome tool for business in general.

Eighteen of the invitees agreed to serve as advisory panel members, and due to my background in computers and a good mind for business, the group elected me as leader of the newly formed panel. I felt honored to be handed the responsibility, and I intended to put my heart into doing whatever I could to ensure the success of this company and the real estate agents who would utilize its services. Before I left Seattle, I heard the company's Wall Street investment banker tell the president to "give Scislow whatever he needs." He wanted to ensure the company remained open to my ideas and those of the panel members. Needless to say, I left Seattle with some pretty high hopes.

Over the next few weeks, many of the attendees made decisions with respect to investing in the company's stock. My personal decision was to invest a sizable amount. I was not alone in this, as other panel members invested handsomely as well. In addition, I spoke with family members and close friends about this opportunity. A number of them wanted to invest because they believed in me and my track record of success. As a result of their confidence, thousands of dollars began pouring in from those who were dear to me in order to acquire company stock. Over the next five months, my enthusiasm for the company's product resulted in increased sales both locally and nationally. All subscriber Internet sites were up and running well. Expansion in the technology center was underway. I had booked several speaking and training tours at various locations around the country. I had appointments with several large mortgage companies in town and was preparing an out-of-state presentation for one of the largest banks and mortgage lenders in the nation. The momentum was building, and I envisioned potential financial returns in the millions of dollars.

By mid-August, my first big out-of-town event had finally arrived—the State Realtor's Convention in Kansas City. For years, I had targeted this part of the country for real estate referrals and relocating transferees. I felt right at home and among friends at the convention and was enthusiastic and fired-up about what I was doing. In the midst of my excitement while working the convention floor, I received a call from Seattle. The gentleman on the line was professional and direct, informing me that he was the acting CEO of the company. His instructions were simple, "Pack up and go home. Stop selling. The company is unable to support the sale of any of its products and has been taken over by creditors."

I immediately began making phone calls to my contacts in Seattle in an attempt to confirm the shocking news. It was mid-afternoon, and all of the company phones were down, voice mail was inoperative, and many of the cell phone numbers of key personnel had been disconnected. When I finally reached the company's Wall Street investment banker, he confirmed the unfortunate news and emphasized that the company had been shut down unexpectedly just hours earlier. It had been taken over by creditors and ninety percent of the employees had been fired and police-escorted out of the building earlier that day. He suggested I get out of Kansas City and take the next plane home. My heart sank.

Over the next few days from my office in Minneapolis, I scrambled to obtain information and provide answers for the other advisory panel members who had been calling and emailing, hoping that I might offer a ray of hope in this dire situation. There was nothing good to report. In addition to fielding these calls, I handled numerous calls from real estate agents and business people who had purchased services as a result of my representation of the company. Providing answers to these folks became a very difficult task; I had nothing to offer them other than an ear to listen. It was a very disheartening time. I began to realize that I would never see the thousands of dollars that I had invested in the company. I would never receive the commissions I had earned or be reimbursed for the travel expenses I had incurred. The success I had dreamed about had turned into a nightmare. Worst of all, others had placed their confidence in me and had bought company stock.

This was not only a financial setback but also an emotional one. I felt that I had let others down, and I felt I had been taken advantage of and lied to. I was disappointed in myself. I was totally caught by surprise. *I should have seen it coming,* I thought. Eventually, I realized my mistake; I had no insight—or clue for that matter—about the company's finances. In fact, none of the members of the advisory panel were privy to that information. What we came to learn was that the company simply overspent itself into bankruptcy.

In the midst of this difficult time, I drew strength from a passage of Scripture: *Consider it all joy my brethren, when you encounter various trials, knowing that the testing of your faith produces endurance* (James 1:2-3). There was no question that this was a trial. I felt beaten down. Nothing so devastating had happened to me in years. Everything had been going so well! As a Christian of nearly twenty years, I knew what it meant to stand on God's Word. I simply needed to do that now. I knew I'd get through this, but I needed comfort during the process so I chose to put the matter in God's hands. These verses did not simply say to lean on God for His help, but spoke clearly to me to be joyful during times of trial and to rejoice in difficult moments because my faith would produce endurance.

I did not really know what the *endurance* part of these verses meant, so I simply chose to be joyful and trusted God for the rest.

I recall that the fear, frustration, and hurt quickly dissipated as a result of the choice to be joyful in this time of trial. Although it did not seem to make sense, it worked and was truly amazing! As I spoke with the friends, family, and business people who had invested in the company, I found them to be more understanding than I had anticipated. At a time when I had been devastated by the sudden turn of events, their understanding was very comforting. Before long, I felt the nightmare was behind me. This one was over but, unfortunately, another was on its way.

A PROMISING VENTURE

In July 2000, when everything seemed to be going well with the Seattle dot-com company and huge financial returns seemed imminent, I also stumbled across an opportunity to invest in a start-up company called Venture in my own hometown of Apple Valley, Minnesota. I first became aware of Venture through a close friend who was employed there. There was an awesome new technology that was going to be unveiled—something that had never been offered before. Although the private stock offering period had been closed out just days before, the powers-that-be were offering me the ability to purchase stock because of my connection, and I agreed to check it out.

Venture's primary business plan was to provide custom, high-speed downloading of music onto a compact disc. The customer would select the type of music they desired from a burn station using a computer touch screen. Once the disc capacity was reached and the burn button pressed, a small robot within a Plexiglas case would custom create the compact disc for two-thirds of the cost of a typical CD. Not only did the product seem incredible, the timing for Venture seemed perfect. Throughout much of 2000, Napster and its illegal piracy of music over the Internet was featured in news headlines around the world. Now, with Venture about to be unveiled as a legal alternative to get fast, custom music, it was sure to be a hit right off the bat.

Initially, over one million music titles were to be available for download from Venture's database and a number of record companies had signed on and were ready to participate. Venture was also scheduled to open a 50,000 square-foot facility in September that would be followed by four additional facilities within the next 12 months, including locations in Chicago and New York. These large facilities would each include a restaurant, a bar/lounge, and a family entertainment center in addition to the multitude of burn stations where music could be easily downloaded.

So, based upon all the information I gathered and reviewed about Venture, I felt comfortable moving ahead with an investment because I believed in the product and the people and anticipated handsome financial returns from the Seattle-based company. It appeared that I would easily double or triple my investment, and, in July, I wrote a check for three times the amount that I had invested in the Seattle-based company. By the end of the week, however, Venture's partner, a well-funded, publicly-traded company, suddenly backed out. The officers of Venture decided to forge ahead, but with limited funding coming solely from its investors, and its owners. In my estimation, the concept was still a winner and I remained positive. The grand opening for the first Venture facility was set for Labor Day.

Filled with anticipation, I headed to the 50,000 square-foot facility just a mile and a half from home. I still clearly remember the Disney-like description of fascinating lighting, music, and mechanical animations that I had read about in the prospectus. This was going to be awesome, and I was a big investor in its success! As I entered the facility, my heart sank into my stomach. I was disappointed in what I saw. The facility looked like a huge warehouse with neon-looking lights above banks of computer terminals (the burn stations) scattered around the room. A number of Venture employees wandered around looking clueless, as the Director of Operations ran around trying to determine what went wrong with the robots at a number of the stations. Worse yet, I saw the faces of the few customers that had found their way to this grand opening. Puzzled looks of confusion abounded. "What's this place all about?" some asked. My mind raced with thoughts of frustration, and I wondered who had been in charge of marketing. This grand opening for Venture took place mere weeks after the demise of the Seattle-based dot-com company and thoughts of another financial debacle now surfaced. It was awful.

In less than two months, the first and only Venture facility closed, and the company was buried in over $2 million of debt. All the money employees, their families, their friends, and I had invested in the company was gone. I found myself "0 for 2" in 2000, and the losses from these two companies, coupled with the overall decline of the stock market this year prompted some self-evaluation. Was I somehow living in error? I believed I was living right; my faith was strong and intact, and I had tithed regularly to church. I knew that I had been tremendously blessed as a result of generous donations, yet now it appeared I was giving those blessings back. I was clueless. I remember trying to calculate in my head how many years of selling homes it would take to recoup what was lost in those few short months between two unfortunate investments and the stock market. Earning a sales commission is just part of the equation. There were deductions for business expenses, income taxes, and the cost of living for a family of six. I began to realize it was going to take many sales over a number of years and a lot of hard work to make up for the losses. It was a sobering thought.

I recalled the relief I felt when I stood on the verses from James, and wondered how my faith was being tested. I believed that I was being challenged to trust in the Lord and not in money. Not that I had placed all my trust in money before, but now I was challenged to place ALL my trust in the Lord and NOT in money. I was starting to learn that no matter how much I analyzed the details or terms of an investment, I could not control the outcome. As much as I liked to think I was intelligent enough to make the right choices, I was humbled and reminded that I was not infallible. I was reminded that, *if I place my trust in Him . . . and put Him first . . . then all things will be added to me* [compilation of Proverbs 3:5-6 and Matthew 6:33].

In the midst of these major financial setbacks, and in spite of the fact that my wife was not happy with my investment "expertise", I chose to be joyful. I made it a point to do exactly what the verses in James said I should do, even though it made little sense. I simply said to myself, *On the basis of faith, I will choose not to worry about this. I will trust that God is doing something in my life, and whatever it is, it will be good—period!*

Once I made that conscious choice in my heart, my spirits once again lifted immediately. I quickly gained emotional momentum and began to move forward again. I knew it would simply take time, and I was okay with that. I would need to sell a lot of homes to recover the dollars that were lost, but I'd do it. I had been selling 100 to 200 homes per year for many years—this was what I was good at! I'd simply focus on selling more homes than ever in order to recover from this setback. Little did I know then, but this was exactly where my next challenge would come from—real estate sales!

IT'S TIME TO SELL!

With the disappointing months of August and September behind me, I started the fourth quarter focused on what I did best— selling homes! In the midst of these challenges, I chose to be joyful and faith-filled. I was gaining strength and was ready to get back into the proverbial mode of success. I have never been a quitter, and I was not going to become one now! October, however, did not manifest any success. It was not until late in the month, after having no sales at all, that I realized something *very strange* was going on. What was it? I had attended the usual amount of appointments for October, but nothing had come together. In an average October, I usually sold ten to twelve homes, but not this October. It seemed that every buyer or seller selected another agent, decided to take his or her home off the market, or opted to stop looking. It became very evident that business was fleeing from me!

By this time, I had been selling homes for over fourteen years, and while I had experienced the occasional dry spell in those years, I had never seen a slow down like this. Typically, the slowest month of the year is December, during which I'd sell five to six homes. But no sales in October were unheard of for me, so I persisted, while also working on projects that I reserve for slow times. One thing I have learned over the years in real estate is that whenever activity slows for a period of time, one day it will suddenly pick up again and go right back to normal. This is what I expected for November. Unfortunately, my expectations were a far cry from reality. I sold just two homes that month compared to an average of twelve sales in previous Novembers. I felt something inexplicable was happening.

Just before Thanksgiving, I stopped by the prayer chapel at Hosanna, the church I was attending in Lakeville, Minnesota, in order to find someone to pray for me. As a frequent visitor to the prayer chapel to get prayer, as well as offer prayer, I wanted to know if God was trying to show me something. Everything seemed to be a challenge, especially from a financial standpoint. Would the Lord reveal something to me that would allow me to escape this onslaught of misfortune?

Upon arriving at the prayer chapel, I met several people I knew, and I shared the many bizarre events I had been experiencing. I shared the pain of the financial setbacks and the details of how my real estate sales were suffering. I pointed out that while I remained positive and joyful throughout these trials, I desired to know if God was trying to show me something. I told them I was living out the verses from James 1:2-3; *Consider it all joy when you encounter various trials, knowing that the testing of your faith produces endurance.* I asked them to pray for me so that I might better understand what was happening to me.

Pastor Dave Housholder, one of the pastors of the church, happened to be in the prayer chapel at that moment. After several members of the prayer team prayed for me, Pastor Dave stated, "I am getting a word from the Lord for Jeff." There was a brief pause, and then he said to me, "The Lord is preparing you for difficult times that lie ahead." That was it. I did not know what it meant, but as you will see, those words became a valuable seed that I would draw on for strength and understanding in the weeks ahead.

The Lord is preparing you for difficult times that lie ahead.

The month of December, statistically the slowest in the year for me, proved to be much like the past two months—I only sold one home. A normal December would produce five to six sales, so just one sale indicated that nothing had changed; something strange was still present in my life. When the fourth quarter ended, it went down as the absolute worst in my entire career—just three sales! To make matters worse, one of those sales fell through on the day it was supposed to close, dropping my quarterly numbers to two. In a quarter when real estate was selling normally for other sales associates, it was not for me, and I had been the state's top-selling Realtor over the past decade.

As I sensed the trials of life mounting, I was more determined than ever to stand on the verses in James; I made them personal, and I quoted them day and night. I shared them with my friends at church and in my men's group. Still, I had no idea why I needed to produce endurance, but on the basis of faith, I forged ahead and was soon to be met head on with my biggest challenge yet.

WE'RE OUT OF HERE!

While the fourth quarter of 2000 went down as the worst personal performance in my real estate career, I was fortunate to have three sales people on my real estate team who were making sales. I was grateful to receive a portion of the commission from those sales, and I felt a small sense of financial security due to having this team in place. At the beginning of December, however, that small sense of security evaporated when I was informed that all three were leaving at the end of the month! They made the decision to branch off and start up their *own* sales team. Although this was a bit disheartening, it was not a complete surprise; I had sensed that they might opt to do this someday, but the timing could not have been worse. I accepted their decision and planned for their departure by the end of the month.

Unfortunately, the bad news did not end there. Two days later I learned that my former sales team had made a deal with my full-time assistant. For over four years she had been my right arm in the running of my successful real estate business. I had employed her to take care of all the office details, including the paperwork for my sales team. The team was now stealing her away. I felt betrayed; by the end of the month I'd have no one left in the office but me! Making this bad news even worse, I learned of my assistant's departure a mere week prior to my family and I flying to Cancun, Mexico, for a two-week vacation. *Unbelievable!* I thought, trying to keep my composure in the midst of these most bizarre events.

At that point in time, I began reminding myself that if I was going to trust God in *all* things, then this too was one of those things in which I needed to trust Him. I recalled that I was supposed to consider this a *joyful* trial! *How can I do that?* I grumbled. I decided to do it anyway, since it had proved beneficial in the past. I certainly could not understand what was happening, nor did I have an inkling of *why* it was happening. I just knew it *was* happening and that I was going to focus and stay the course. Above all, I was going to choose to be joyful.

Over the next few days, I pondered what I should do with my business under these confusing circumstances. In a few short days I would leave for vacation and when I returned, my sales team and assistant would be gone. Clearly I had no time to replace my assistant. Should I stay home and cancel the trip? Should I allow my staff to remain in the office while I was out of town? I ultimately decided that they needed to leave before I left town, since I no longer trusted them to consider my best interests in my absence. I informed them that they needed to be out before I left for vacation.

On December 14, the day before flying to Cancun, everyone had left. I forwarded the phones to voice mail and locked the doors to my office, a painful experience. At the last minute, I again considered canceling the trip. *I need to get another assistant hired immediately,* I thought to myself. I needed a new sales team, and I needed to start selling some homes. So many immediate to-dos congested my thinking. My mind was racing and there was an uneasy heaviness wanting to consume me.

Eventually, I realized that canceling our vacation would not be fair to my kids, my wife, or me. Staying home was simply not an option; we flew out bright and early on December 15. During the flight, I reflected on the past few months. It became increasingly clear that *something extremely bizarre* was going on. I did not understand it, I could not explain it, and I did not have any control over it. My faith was being tested big time. I knew this. It had become clearer than ever. In those moments, I consciously decided to meet any *new* challenge head on, and with faith and trust in God's Word, I would overcome whatever came my way.

During our vacation, I praised God. I thanked Him for what He was doing, although I had no clue what it was. I continued to draw strength from Pastor Dave's word of knowledge; I was being prepared for difficult times that lie ahead. But at the same time, I thought to myself, *Haven't I encountered enough difficult times already? How much more difficult could things get?* Little did I know, but the difficulties were only beginning, and the magnitude of challenge was still on the way. How true the pastor's words would prove to be!

TAKE THE MONEY AND RUN

For two wonderful weeks, my family and I enjoyed the warmth of the Mexican sunshine and refreshing ocean surf. This was our tenth visit to Cancun and one that I most desperately needed. We had escaped the frigid Minnesota winter briefly and spent time with close friends with whom we vacationed each year in Cancun. It was so rewarding not to spend that time worrying about the unfortunate situation waiting for me back home. Once again, I noticed that by turning my problems over to the Lord, and by praising Him in times of difficulty, I made it through the trial just fine. I saw a clear pattern and was amazed by it.

As often happens on vacation, time passed quickly, and once back home, reality began to set in. I needed to re-open the office, hire an administrative assistant, and build a sales team. When my wife and I were married in 1987, she got her real estate license and worked as my office administrator. For nine years we worked together before she chose to stay at home with our children, at which point I hired the assistant who had just left with my sales team. My wife had maintained an active real estate license, and it was a true blessing when she said she'd come back to work in the office until I could find a new licensed assistant.

While January is typically a quiet real estate month in the Twin Cities, this one started out well for me. I put together six sales—three times as many sales as I had the entire fourth quarter of 2000! This was excellent! I felt I was getting back on track. Then another bombshell dropped. Near the end of January, I realized that I had not received an expected paycheck from my RE/MAX broker—my portion of the commission on a sale transacted by a former sales team member while he was on my team. After some inquiries, I learned that the sale had not been reported properly. It had, in fact, been reported as a sale independent of my 'team.' In other words, I would not be receiving the portion of the commission I was due per the written contract with my former team member. Believing this was a simple mistake, I asked the broker to speak with the former team member about this sale and the commission that I failed to receive. Within a couple days, the broker got back to me and informed me that the former team member felt the commission belonged solely to him! It was clear to me that this sale was transacted prior to his departure and within the timeframe of our contract.

I became suspicious and searched each listing the sales team had on the books when they were part of my team. Several additional listings of theirs had been sold immediately prior to their departure. Since these sales were made while I was their team leader I deserved a portion of those commissions. Once again I found myself dealing with an issue of disappearing money. I could not believe it. I had trusted these people. In fact, I had once even considered making one of the sales team members a partner, or selling the business to the team someday. Now we were arguing over commission splits. I was personally devastated and could not understand why this was happening.

Since the broker was unable to mediate a solution, thousands of dollars from the contested sales that had not yet closed would be held in the broker's escrow account until the matter was settled. The broker told me that I had the option of pursuing this matter in court, so I obtained a legal opinion from an attorney who stated that the contract was clear and well-written. He felt I would prevail and win a judgment in court for the commissions in question if I chose to pursue this. I needed time to consider what I should do. Even with the likelihood of winning in court, was I up for suing my former team for money? Was that the right thing to do? They were waiting for my first move.

In the midst of yet another incredible setback I reminded myself, *I need to stay focused, and joyful. These events are beyond my comprehension, but I am up for the challenge. Praise God!* After much thought and prayer, I opted to write a letter to the sales team giving them the opportunity to search their hearts and act upon what they felt was right. I felt the Lord leading me in that direction, and in order for this letter to be genuine, I needed to be willing to accept whatever they chose to do. They obviously felt the money belonged to them. I stated in my letter that I would abide by whatever they felt their hearts were telling them, and that if they felt the money truly belonged to them, they could use the letter as their ticket to have all the money held in escrow released to them. I stated that I would not pursue them in court and that I trusted them to do what was right.

Now, this was a very difficult letter for me to write. I felt the thousands of commission dollars were unmistakably mine through a clearly spelled out contract and that I simply needed to claim it legally. Since I had lost a small fortune between the business failures, plummeting stock market, and the worst quarter in my real estate career, I really needed the money! Throughout all this deliberation, I sensed God telling me to send the letter. I heard Him saying to forgive them and not to worry about money or anything else. So, I sent the letter to the sales team and sent a copy to my broker.

Nearly a week went by without a reply, at which point I contacted my broker and inquired if he had heard anything from the sales team. He had not, but indicated he would call and solicit their response. Later that day the broker called me back. He stated the sales team's response: "We're all glad that this matter has been resolved." They kept the money, and I was shocked! At this point I became more concerned about the series of events that were happening than the events themselves. Why did I keep encountering such completely out-of-the-ordinary events? It was clear I was in the middle of something very strange, but I could not figure it out. It simply made no sense. I was beginning to feel like Job of the Old Testament but caught myself and thought, *No, I'm not Job*. In each peculiar and frustrating instance, as I searched deep in my heart to find joy in the midst of these challenges, the Lord got me through each bump in the road, with an outcome that was better than I expected. *This is no time to change that approach*, I thought.

It really is difficult to express how strange it seems to praise God in the middle of troubled times. But somehow, according to those verses in the first chapter of James, my faith was being tested in order to produce what would prove to be much-needed endurance. I searched for more answers in Scripture and found some specific verses from 1 Peter 4:12-13: *. . . do not be surprised at the fiery ordeal among you, which comes upon you for your testing, as though some strange thing were happening to you; but to the degree that you share the sufferings of Christ, keep on rejoicing; so that also at the revelation of His glory, you may rejoice with exultation.* Some strange thing seemed to me like an understatement, but I saw hope in these verses. I envisioned the revelation of God's glory as the breakthrough and victory over these trials! It would be a time for me to rejoice in exultation. I believed that and proceeded on the basis of faith.

CHAPTER 2

— A Blow to the Body —

CHAPTER 2

I was glad to have January behind me, for it was a period of considerable emotional pain. As I focused more on getting my office up and running again, the personal hurt subsided. As February arrived, I took a big breath and looked back over the past six months. I reflected on the avalanche of setbacks that threatened to overtake me; but two thoughts continued to resonate with me: First, life had to start improving soon, and second, I was determined to get things back on track.

I pressed on, but before the first week of the month came to a close, I began feeling like I had the stomach flu. The symptoms included slight fever, loss of appetite, nausea, and lack of motivation. After about a week and a half of this persistent ill-feeling, I opted to visit the local clinic seeking some antibiotic or other quick fix to help me feel better. As soon as the doctor saw me, he said I showed signs of having hepatitis. I knew very little about hepatitis, simply that it was not good. I learned that it meant 'enlarged liver' and that something may have caused my liver to become inflamed. It was not long before I began to think, *Difficult times . . . Now even my health is under attack!*

The doctor ordered blood tests to determine if my body had produced any known hepatitis antibodies that would enable the doctors to identify the type of hepatitis that I had apparently contracted. These initial tests were looking for types A, B, and C. The results did not confirm hepatitis at all. I was asked to return for additional tests over the next few days. On February 16, I was tested again for hepatitis A, B, and C. By this time the doctor was even more certain that I had hepatitis based on physical observation, but to his amazement, each test came back negative! I was showing all the signs of hepatitis, but it could not be proven. This was puzzling for everyone.

Along with the antibody tests, my enzyme counts were tested to determine if I, in fact, had any liver damage. These tests revealed that my liver was under attack and had experienced some fairly severe damage. The doctor at the clinic immediately indicated that I was in need of a specialist. After a few phone calls, I had the name of the best hepatitis doctor in the Twin Cities area. My local doctor made the appropriate referral, and I was given a prompt appointment with the specialist. Within a few days, I was in the specialist's office where, upon seeing me, he agreed that I had some form of hepatitis. He began ordering a number of tests to determine which type I had contracted. He retested for types A, B, and C and proceeded to test for D and E. Some tests were sent to local hospitals, others to the University of Minnesota, and one was sent to the CDC (Center for Disease Control) in Atlanta, Georgia. With all these blood tests going on, I was beginning to feel like a pincushion; at one sitting I recall the nurse drawing eleven tubes of blood!

The first test results to return were for types A, B, and C. Just as with the clinic's findings, results returned negative. At this point the specialist began thinking my liver might be under attack by a parasite so he scheduled me for an abdominal CAT scan the next day. This test also proved to be negative in all respects. Within a few days, the other hepatitis tests returned negative as well. In just three weeks, my weight had fallen from 169 to 158 pounds. I was not hungry and felt weak and very sick. I had to force myself to eat. My skin was yellow and my urine bright orange.

From what I was being told, I found out that most of those who contract (acute) hepatitis A recover. The other types of hepatitis are oftentimes chronic and result in death over the long term. In my case, they pretty much concluded that I had contracted a new or undetectable form of hepatitis. As a result, they could not provide any sort of prognosis as to what I might expect by way of an outcome. I felt my faith being tested to a greater degree than ever before, even in light of the past six months. This time it was my health—my very existence! My physical state was terrible, weak, and sickly. Emotionally, I was wrestling with depression, one of the common symptoms of hepatitis because the patient feels physically incapable of doing anything.

Still, although my physical and emotional states were experiencing quite a battle, my spiritual side was strong and focused. There was no question that something extremely unusual had been going on in my life way beyond my ability to explain or identify. Each time I considered the trial to be joyful and praised God in the midst of it, I found myself getting over the hurdle instead of letting it get the best of me. As a result, I was more determined than ever to meet this current challenge head on with joy and faith in my heart.

MARCH 1, 2001, BLOOD TEST RESULTS

⊠ Fairview Clinics

Dear ___Jeff Scislow___

DOB _____ Phone No. _____

_____ Date of Test
__3-1-01__ Date Sent
__cS__ Initials

The following tests were checked recently and the results noted below.

*Test explanations are brief and do not reflect all diagnostic uses.

Normal	Abnormal	
☐	☐	**Glucose** _____
		• A screening test for diabetes
☐	☐	**Glycosylated hemoglobin** _____ %
		Average blood glucose _____
		• Long-term check of average blood sugar
		3-6% or less = excellent control or non-diabetic
		6-8% = good control
		9-14% = poor control
☐	☐	**Kidney tests/Electrolytes**
		• Checks how well the kidneys are working and measures body salts which may be affected by medications.
☐	☐	**Liver tests**
		• Checks how well the liver is functioning
☐	☐	**Thyroid tests**
		• Checks thyroid function and body metabolism
☑	☐	**CBC/Hgb** _____
		• Complete blood cell count (notes presence of infection, anemia, etc.) and checks the number and appearance of blood components and cells.
☑	☐	**Hemoglobin** 15.4 g/dL [N= 13.7 to 17.5]
		• Checks the oxygen-carrying capacity of the blood
☐	☐	**Urinalysis**
		• Checks for urine abnormalities such as infection, blood or sugar
☐	☐	**PSA**
		• Prostate screening test for abnormal antigens
☐	☐	**Hemoccult**
		• Checks for presence of blood in stool
☐	☐	**H. Pylori - Stomach Bacteria**
☑	☐	**Other** Hep A Antibody total ⊖ (sign of side acwcation)
☑	☐	**Other** Hep A IgM antibody ⊖ (sign of acute infection)
☑		**Other** Hep B core antibody ⊖

(4/22/01)

LIPID PROFILE	Desirable	Borderline	Your Result
Cholesterol	Less than 200	200-240	
HDL "Good Chol"	Greater than 35	--	
LDL "Bad Chol"	Less than 130	130-160	
Triglycerides	Below 200	200-400	

Medical Imaging Results / X-Ray

Normal	Abnormal	
☐	☐	X-ray(s) of _____
☐	☐	Mammogram
☐	☐	Ultrasound
☐	☐	Dexascan

Comments:	12/6/00	2/16/01	2/19/01	2/23	2/29	4/26
[N=0-70]←→ ALT	47	3454	3595	3278	—	2021
[N=0-55]←→ AST	29	1902	2174	1805	—	1356
[N=0-16]←→ Total Bil	0.8	—	—	11.8	—	19.8
INR	[N= 0.8 to 1.2]			2.9	1.5	1.3

☐ Make follow-up appointment with provider.
☐ Make follow-up appointment for labs.

☐	**No further action is necessary.**

☐   Comments and recommended follow up: _____

_____

Please make a follow up appointment if you have additional questions.

Sincerely,

By the first week of March, the specialist confessed, "I am sorry, but we cannot determine what type of hepatitis you have nor do we really know how you contracted it. We can't say for sure how long it will take to recover, or for that matter, whether you *will* recover. You have a good attitude and I have a hunch you will come through this and have a full recovery, but not for at least six months." The specialist scheduled me for weekly blood testing and monitoring. By mid-March I began to feel better and acquired a desire for food once again. My lack of appetite had caused my weight to drop all the way to 156 pounds.

On a positive note, my weekly visit to the specialist on March 15 revealed that my "enzyme levels" had dropped down from their astronomically dangerous levels. I was quite excited about the improvement, and my emotional state quickly improved after hearing this good news. My spiritual state remained strong as I again considered this challenging trial joyful, knowing that the testing of my faith was producing endurance. Endurance for what, I still did not know. It would soon be revealed however, as I proceeded down the path of encountering a person's worst nightmare.

WHY ME?

The tsunami of bizarre events that I had experienced over the past six months had taken a financial toll, an emotional toll, and now a physical one. I was also taken to the limit of my wits at times, but I continued to trust in the Lord—that He had some light at the end of this dark tunnel. I persisted in rejoicing in the face of these trials. Although weakened by hepatitis, the last half of March found me venturing out, taking listings, and selling homes again. I was optimistic that I would be able to recoup all that was lost, no matter how long it took. The financial devastation we had experienced was incredible, but now that my health seemed to be improving, I was motivated to turn things around financially. During the last two weeks of March, business began improving. I listed six homes and sold eight!

Just as things seemed to be taking a positive turn, while sitting at my desk, I felt a slight trickle from my nose. Thinking nothing of it, I wiped it with the back of my finger and realized it was blood! *What in the world?* I thought, *I don't get nosebleeds.* I worked to get the bleeding under control and concluded it had resulted from an overly dry office environment. I immediately went out and purchased a portable humidifier hoping it would help. Over the next few days, I noticed my face breaking out. It progressed rapidly over the next week until I had large pimples all over my face. Boils developed, even on my forehead. My face swelled. It was red, puffy, and very sore. I had also developed an aggressive cough. I tried lozenges and syrups but to no avail. I started getting headaches from the progressive coughing. I prayed persistently during this time, asking God to show me what was happening.

At the end of March, I went to the hospital emergency room where the doctor determined that I was battling tracheitis, a condition in which my trachea was inflamed with a possible infection, the result of a virus going around. He prescribed the antibiotic Doxycycline and sent me home. I said to myself, *I've always been a healthy person. What's happening to me?* I simply wanted to be healthy so I could focus on working and replenishing the financial resources that had been stripped away.

My spiritual side was questioning these trying circumstances as well. Not only did I wonder *what* was going on, I wondered *why*. Although I wanted to continue to trust God under all circumstances, I did wonder *Why me?* from time to time. I made a very conscious effort not to blame God for what was happening. I simply looked to Him as the One who could help me through it and trusted Him to do that. I knew that I might never know fully why this was happening, but I did have a sense that I would come to a better understanding of it at some point.

My world was spinning, and everything was happening all at once. Not only was my nose bleeding off and on during the day and night, but, as I coughed more, blood also began to accompany the coughing. In the mornings, I was peeling dried blood from my gums, and I became embarrassed to be seen in public with my face so broken out from the acne and the boils and my eyes so yellow from the effects of the hepatitis. The Doxycycline was not working. My kids wondered what was wrong with daddy. I was coughing harder and more frequently. My headaches worsened, and my eyes began to ache. I noticed my vision had begun to grow dim. I found it difficult to read and identify road signs as I traveled in the car. I felt totally overwhelmed and completely exhausted. I did not even consider that something might be seriously wrong, I simply concluded that I was just tired, stressed, and in need of some catch-up sleep. My main concern was my facial appearance, so I paid much less attention to my dimming vision or the other symptoms.

Before going to bed on April 1, I heard the Lord speak to my heart in an ever-so-small voice. He told me to stop taking a particular product that I had begun taking two weeks earlier. He said it was causing an allergic reaction that was producing the acne and the boils on my face. I stopped using it at once. Amazingly, over the next couple of days, I saw a complete turnaround as my face began to clear up. "Hallelujah!" I cried with much enthusiasm! Then, a few mornings later, I woke and noticed a lump on my tongue. I quickly went to the mirror and, to my horror, saw a black-colored, pea-sized lump right in the middle of my tongue! Evidently, the lozenge that I had been sucking on for my sore throat and cough had cut my tongue while I was sleeping. This black coloring was the dried blood that had filled up inside my tongue! I looked at myself in the mirror and then looked to heaven and shouted, "God! What is going on?

I have been faithful! Is there something I need to do that I am not doing? What is going on, Lord?"

It was hard to digest all that was happening in my life. It was truly mind-boggling. After a few minutes, I regained my composure and once again made the choice to stand on God's Word no matter what. But when would this all conclude? When would my *joyful* trials come to an end? I thought about how other people might handle similar situations, and, as my thoughts bounced around on how to respond to these back-to-back challenges, my mind was set at ease as I remembered Psalm 34:19; *Many are the afflictions of the righteous, but the Lord delivers him out of them all.*

Wow, I thought, *Isn't that the truth!* I offered up a brief prayer, "Thank You, Lord, for what You are doing. I'm Yours, and I know that You have a plan. Although I have no idea what it is, I will trust You and give You thanks for being there for me! I trust that, *all things are going to work together for good*, according to Romans 8:28—hallelujah!"

THE DIVINE APPOINTMENT

On April 5, I received a phone call in the morning from a past real estate client. She said, "Jeff, I heard you've been sick. Our pastor is in town today but is leaving for Arizona tomorrow. He has an incredible gift of healing. I asked him if he would be willing to pray for you, and he said he would. How does 7:00 p.m. tonight sound, at our church on Lake Street in Minneapolis? I think it is a divine appointment." At this point I wanted all the prayer I could get and agreed to the meeting. My wife and our neighbor Terri accompanied me to the church that night. Terri wanted to receive prayer as well, since she had been battling pneumonia for weeks.

We met my past client at the entrance to the church. Once inside, we were introduced to Pastor Holmes. We proceeded to his pastoral office. We each took a seat and began sharing our prayer requests. First he prayed for Terri and then for me, and he asked the Lord to heal us of our respective illnesses—Terri's pneumonia and my hepatitis, coughing, bleeding, etc. His prayers for us lasted about three to five minutes each. Toward the end of his prayer for me I experienced something quite unique—something I can best explain as a vision.

During the prayer, for a period of approximately forty-five seconds, I saw what best resembled a video clip. It was a vivid trip through the inside of a human body, as if it was being viewed with a fiber optic internal camera. After a brief moment, I sensed it was *my* body. I saw five or six white lights that appeared only as dots. They were moving at what I might call the speed of light, and in all directions, leaving comet-like tails behind them! The clear visual image I was seeing continued through many parts of my body. These little white lights raced all over, down tubes, and past my heart and other organs. The pink and red colors of the blood, the tissue, and the organs were all so real. The instant the prayer ended so did the vision.

I shared this with everyone in the room. No one knew what it meant. I only knew that the vision had something to do with the inside of my body. I did not think much more of the vision that night.

As we headed home, Terri indicated she was feeling 100 percent better. The ravaging cough that accompanied her on the way to the church had subsided. It came to pass that she was miraculously healed that night. I, on the other hand, continued coughing all the way home. I did not feel any different nor were there any signs of improvement in me. I did not realize at that time, however, that I had just been on a divine appointment—one that would soon manifest into an incredible miracle.

AFTER YOU SUFFER

As we drove home from receiving prayer at the church, I grew very tired. The challenging events that I had been facing were taking their toll on me. I had recently been waking in the middle of the night coughing and had found it difficult to get a good night's rest, reasonably explaining why I had felt so run down and tired during the past couple of weeks. As soon as we got home, I went straight to bed, hoping for a good night's rest. Once again, however, I was awakened by the cough in the middle of the night.

At 4:00 a.m. I went down to the kitchen to get a banana, which seemed like the best food for my sore throat. I grabbed the television controller and began flipping through the channels. I landed on a late night channel that had a Bible verse displayed on the screen. It seemed to JUMP OUT at me. As I read it, it came to life! It was my verse! It explained what I had been going through. It was as if I was awakened from my sleep in order to see this verse: *After you have suffered a little while, the God of all grace, who called you to His eternal glory in Christ, shall Himself, restore, strengthen, perfect, establish and confirm you* (1 Peter 5:10).

After you have suffered a little while, the God of all grace, who called you to His eternal glory in Christ, shall Himself, restore, strengthen, perfect, establish and confirm you.

After reading this I responded, "That's me, Lord. I sure have been suffering!" In the midst of my excitement over seeing this very specific verse on TV, at this exact point in time in the middle of the night, my thoughts gravitated to the restoration, strengthening, and perfecting part of that verse. I sensed that the Lord had heard all my prayers and that He was about to deliver me from all the trials, tribulations, and terrible situations I had been going through for many months. Somehow, He was going to issue me a passing grade on all my tests! Right smack in the middle of my enthusiasm, in an instant of time, I heard the Lord speak to my heart with these very clear and direct words: *There is more to come.*

But, Lord, no . . . not more, I immediately thought to myself.

There is more to come.

I had no idea what *more* meant, but it seemed as if I was being prepared for the *more*; and in a way I was actually looking forward to it because I knew God would get me through it. Sure, I wanted all this to be over, but I felt strong enough to continue on this most amazing journey. I was determined to get through whatever bizarre situation I encountered, knowing there would be a good outcome in the end. I knew this to be true: *I can do all things through Christ who strengthens me.*

—PHILIPPIANS 4:13

SOME SWEET R & R

The day after I was prayed for, after getting the okay from my wife, I chose to check into a local motel to get some needed rest and relaxation. I knew that two days of no work, no phones, no kids, no pets, and an indoor swimming pool, sauna, and Jacuzzi would do wonders for me. The first night was wonderful. The classic, lay back, and do-nothing evening included an in-the-room Jacuzzi and movie before retiring early. I scored about nine hours of rest that night, the longest in recent history for me. Even with that much sleep, I still felt tired and completely worn out once I awoke. As I lay in bed, I concluded that I had just been through so much that it would take more than one night's rest to get me feeling normal again. I looked forward to my second relaxing day of lounging around the pool, doing nothing, and going to bed early.

As I got out of bed and stood up, I felt rather dizzy and lightheaded. *Perhaps, I have an ear infection without the pain,* I thought, knowing that ear infections could affect one's balance. In a phone call to my wife, I relayed this sense of dizziness to her, and after experiencing so many strange events recently, she was not taking any chances. She offered to pick me up and drive me to the local clinic in Eagan, Minnesota, to have me checked out. I agreed.

YOU'RE REALLY, REALLY SICK

Upon seeing the doctor at the clinic, he suggested a blood test based on my appearance and description of symptoms. In a few minutes the results were back. The doctor returned with a concerned look on his face—very concerned. He wanted to bring my wife into the room, and I immediately got a sense that more bad news was on the way. My wife and I sat next to each other, and the doctor sat facing us. He took a deep breath, and with sad, compassion-filled eyes said, "I don't know how to tell you this, but you're really, really sick." He went on to say, "Your blood levels are extremely low, and I am going to recommend immediate ambulance transport to the hospital."

When asked which hospital I preferred, I responded, "Burnsville Ridges," since it was the closest facility from my home. He stated, "Burnsville will not have the facilities that you are going to need," and suggested either Fairview Southdale in Edina or United Hospital in St. Paul. His response did not provide any sense of comfort. We wrestled briefly with the doctor about not wanting to be driven in the ambulance; we preferred to drive ourselves. He cautiously agreed and offered the following words of warning: "Don't trip or fall, drive slowly, and, whatever you do, do not get into an accident."

On Saturday, April 7, 2001, at 5:00 p.m., we departed from the clinic in Eagan and headed to United Hospital in St. Paul where the greatest battle of all would begin—the battle for my life! In the days that lay ahead, the limits of my faith would be tested beyond anything I could imagine, and my need for endurance would never be greater!

THE EMERGENCY ROOM

As we drove to the emergency room, both my wife and I were scared. What was wrong with me? What did the blood test reveal that alarmed the doctor so much? What was going to happen? What should I do now? My wife began to pray, and we both got on our cell phones and began calling everyone we knew to request prayer. We called family, friends, church members, and our pastors. We even called friends as far away as Jamaica and Australia. A number of people who lived in town jumped in their cars and headed to the hospital to meet us.

I remember quoting Bible verses out loud—every verse I could think of that provided a promise and a defense, particularly: *Greater is He who is in me, than he who is in the world* (1 John 4:4); *No weapon formed against me shall prosper* (Isaiah 54:17); and *God has not given me a spirit of fear, but of love, power and a sound mind* (2 Timothy 1:7). I kept calling on the Lord, through His Word, to direct my thoughts and to help me. I had no idea what was going on. The one thing I knew for sure was that it was very serious!

Upon arriving at the emergency room, they checked me in and drew more blood. I had become somewhat used to having blood drawn since I had been tested regularly during the bout with hepatitis. The blood tests came back, and the results were shocking; all three major components of my blood were at basement levels.

My hemoglobin (red cells), which are responsible for carrying oxygen to the muscles, brain, and entire body, were so low that they immediately ordered a blood transfusion. My blood platelets, which are responsible for blood clotting, were so low that they ordered a platelet transfusion. My white cell count, which is indicative of the immune system's capability, was so low that I had virtually no immune system and was highly susceptible to any foreign invader such as bacteria, virus, or fungus. A common cold could kill me! Worse yet, white cells cannot be transfused since they only have a life span of a few days once they are produced in the body. The ER staff immediately began an intravenous flow of antibiotics to provide protection from potential bacteria that could kill me.

As I lay in the emergency room, having a number of tubes and needles stuck in both my hands and arms, I stared at the ceiling and thought to myself, *This is my life; unbelievable.* I had come to a point where I had stopped wondering *what* was happening; it was not possible to comprehend. I then began to recall once again all the crazy events that I had experienced over the past year and thought to myself, *This is just the next thing in a string of unfortunate and bizarre happenings. No matter what I am about to go through, I will conquer it and it will not conquer me. God is with me and He is greater than any problem I will ever face.*

Over the next few hours, a number of concerned family and friends arrived at the hospital to encourage, comfort, and pray for me. Even as a tough former Marine that was determined to get through this, the emotions of fear and uncertainty continued with their unrelenting assault. These visitors, who dropped what they were doing and came to stand beside me in the emergency room on that Saturday night, played a very significant role in my life. Not only did they supply encouragement and prayerful support, but, by being there for me, they also established an assurance of their ongoing support, the support I would need for what was just around the corner—the battle of, and for, my life!

CHAPTER 3

— TWENTY-EIGHT DAYS IN THE HOSPITAL —

*The Lord is my shepherd. I shall not want. He makes me lie
down in green pastures. He leads me beside quiet waters.
He restores my soul. He guides me in paths of righteousness for
His name's sake. Even though I walk through the valley of the
shadow of death, I will fear no evil, for You are with me;
Your rod and Your staff, they comfort me.*
—PSALM 23:1–4

CHAPTER 3

SUNDAY, APRIL 8

I woke early in my new environment—a hospital bed in the oncology ward at United Hospital in St. Paul. I had lost fourteen pounds over the past couple of months and was not looking or feeling my best, and now I was in the hospital. The night before, in the emergency room, the doctors had run a number of tests on me. They followed those tests with several blood transfusions to increase my low blood levels. During the course of this day, I would meet three different doctors to discuss the results further.

The first doctor to visit came with results from tests done on my liver. I had told them about my bout with hepatitis the previous month, so they also ran a series of tests to evaluate my liver functions. The hepatitis specialist I had been seeing in February and March had indicated it would be six months before my liver function might return to normal. Well, the tests results blew that projection away—they came back completely normal—in just three weeks my sick and ailing liver functions had been restored to completely normal levels!

The second doctor to pay a visit was an oncologist, and he informed me that they did not know for certain with what I had been stricken. He told me that there was a possibility that a virus, such as the one that had most likely attacked my liver, was now suppressing my bone marrow production. On the other hand, it could be something more serious, such as leukemia or aplastic anemia. Only a bone marrow biopsy would determine which situation I was facing, and one was scheduled for me very early the following day.

The third doctor to visit me was an internal medicine specialist. His visit was more one of curiosity and amazement. In my conversation with him, he asked me if I had suffered from any recent bleeding. I let him know that about three weeks earlier I had experienced bleeding from my nose, gums, and face and that I was also coughing it up, although it had completely stopped just three days ago. That was the part he could not figure out—why the bleeding stopped when it should have grown worse. He informed me that the bleeding had probably begun due to a low platelet count—a count which had fallen to just 2,000 when admitted to the hospital (normal platelet counts range from 130,000 to 430,000). He simply could not understand why there were no signs of internal bleeding, a symptom on its own that could have caused my death. He concluded that it was medically impossible for the bleeding to have started three weeks ago, for my platelet count to diminish to near non-existence, and for the bleeding to have stopped three days ago without any signs of internal bleeding.

It was only after this conversation that it began to dawn on me that something miraculous had occurred after receiving prayer from Pastor Holmes just three days prior. Something took place inside my body when all those little white lights were racing around inside. Although I had the privilege of seeing this vision during the prayer, I did not fully understand the impact of that prayer until this day.

MONDAY, APRIL 9

BONE MARROW BIOPSY

The pinnacle of my day was a bone marrow biopsy. I knew it would not be a pleasant experience, but I geared up for it, knowing it would bring me one step closer to a diagnosis and (hopefully) an understanding of what was going on with me. At 10 a.m., the pathologist and his team arrived and began the procedure with an IV of morphine, followed by an incision. Next, they drilled and removed a small cylinder of hip bone and inserted a large needle into the opening of my hip in an attempt to draw out some bone marrow for testing. Needless to say, this was an uncomfortable process.

Gabriel Outside My Door

Later in the afternoon, the morphine had worn off, and I was feeling the pain. About that time, I received a phone call from Pat Moe, one of the pastors from our church. She had visited me the day before and spent some time praying with me in my room. She called to convey an absolutely amazing message. Recalling her time in my hospital room, she said, "The glory of the Lord was extremely strong yesterday. I have visited many, many people in hospitals before but have only experienced the presence and glory of God one other time like I did while in your room. On that other occasion, God miraculously healed that person, and I believe He is going to heal you too."

"Awesome! Praise God! I believe that too!" was my response.

She continued, "But that's not all. As I left your room, I saw an eight-foot angel standing in the hall next to your door, as if he was guarding it. He appeared to be dressed in some type of battle gear. As I walked toward the elevator, I prayed and asked God what I had just seen. God said, 'That is Gabriel.'"

For a moment I was stunned and shocked. Then I replied, "Praise the Lord! Psalm 34:7 says, *The angel of the Lord encamps around those who fear Him, and rescues them!* Wow! I am going to be rescued!" This vision and these words from Pastor Moe, which God planned for me to hear at that exact time, were awesome. They gave me the strength I would need after receiving the diagnosis.

Retinal Hemorrhaging

As if I had not had enough excitement for the day already, I was also scheduled to see an ophthalmologist in order to determine why my vision had dimmed so significantly. Upon examination, he discovered that the low blood counts and profuse coughing had caused blood vessels in the back of my retinas to burst. While the bleeding had stopped, scar tissue was preventing light from properly passing within my eye. As a result, I had an obscured spectrum of sight. I was unable to read a book if I looked straight at it. My vision was improved slightly if I looked out of the corner of my eyes rather than straight ahead. The ophthalmologist predicted that my vision would clear up in approximately four months as I continued to receive blood transfusions.

Tuesday, April 10
Biopsy Results

I will never forget Tuesday, April 10, 2001. Could you imagine forgetting the day your doctor informed you that you had a disease that would likely take your life? I remember the moment vividly. It was mid-morning. The lights in the room were dim like the moment I was about to experience.

In walked the oncologist with his clipboard and a mundane expression. His initial words were simple and to the point, "Well, you have aplastic anemia."

I knew what this meant! It was awful! I had read about it on-line, and immediately my heart felt like a molten cup of lead burning deeply as it spilled into the depths of my gut. I felt the most unusual and uncomfortable shift in my body's chemistry, like a gripping, dry heat that was engulfing my total existence and sucking the life out of me. I had never felt anything so uncomfortable in my life.

It seemed like a bad dream, and seconds like an eternity. My thoughts raced in multiple directions. One instant I was hit with fear, the next I fought for internal composure. I thought of my family—no husband, no daddy. I had never thought so fast before in my life! Then, I realized I had a choice to make right then and there—in my mind and deep within my very soul. Would I be ruled by fear or by faith? Would I focus on my circumstances or on God's promises of healing? God had brought me through a year's worth of challenges thus far, and I sensed that He had prepared me for this very time. My all-knowing God knew that this disease would attack me at this particular time in my life, and He had been strengthening me to meet it head on. On top of all this, He had Gabriel standing outside my door! Why should I be fearful?

Within seconds of my mental sabbatical, in a room filled with silence, I propped myself up in my bed, looked the oncologist straight in the eye, and, with a smile on my face and a heart of determination, said, "Wow! Won't this make a great testimony when God heals me!"

The oncologist was shocked at my remark and proceeded to explain the serious nature of the diagnosis. He pointed out that my diagnosis fell into the category of "severe" aplastic anemia, one much worse than most. The severity was due to my low blood numbers and the fact no marrow stem cells were found during the biopsy— both of these factors reduced the chances of successful treatment.

WHAT IS APLASTIC ANEMIA?

Aplastic anemia is an autoimmune disease where the immune system attacks the bone marrow. Since the immune system is made up of white cells and the bone marrow produces virtually all blood cells, including the white cells, aplastic anemia is in essence a disease that causes the immune system to commit suicide. Once the disease kills the bone marrow, the body is incapable of producing blood cells that are needed to sustain life.

Aplastic anemia can be linked to several factors such as radiation, environmental toxins, and hepatitis. Although the doctors could not be certain why I had contracted the disease, they speculated that the bout with hepatitis set off the aplastic anemia. The likelihood of hepatitis triggering aplastic anemia in a human body is roughly one in three million according to the oncologist, and the disease itself is extremely rare, with only 496 reported cases throughout the United States in 2000.

TWO MEDICAL OPTIONS

I learned from the oncologist that people with aplastic anemia have two possible treatment options. The first option, which is always preferred, is a treatment called ATG (anti-thymocyte globulin). The second option, and usually the last resort, is a bone marrow transplant. Even though I was forty-four years old with a history of good health and physical condition, the doctor was not optimistic that I would survive a bone marrow transplant. The odds were simply against it. He also discussed with me whether or not to even try the first option since my bone marrow biopsy had come back showing neither marrow nor stem cells. And for the treatment to have a chance of success, marrow stem cells would need to be present. Before proceeding with the first option, my biopsy was immediately reviewed by a team of specialists at the University of Minnesota Bone Marrow Transplant Center, and, upon their review, the doctors concluded there was nothing to lose by attempting the ATG treatment. If successful, a partial increase in my blood levels would appear in approximately two weeks. Believe it or not, the ATG treatment involved running horse blood through my body in a series of eight transfusions. The procedure was scheduled to commence on the evening of April 11.

The doctors made it clear to me, however, that even if my blood levels notched up a bit as a result of the ATG treatment, they would never return to normal levels due to the degree of damage that had been done. Additionally, if any marrow stem cells undetected by the biopsy did remain, they would be insufficient to produce enough blood cells to return the blood counts to normal levels. They wanted me to understand that the prognosis was not good and my chance for survival was slim.

WEDNESDAY, APRIL 11

DAILY ROUTINE

In my attempt to stay focused on whatever I would face in the days ahead, I followed a daily routine. First thing in the morning, of course, was my visit with the nurse and her blood cart. Each day I deposited two or three, sometimes even five, tubes of blood for testing. Each morning the oncologist would pop his head in the door with the results and ask me how I was doing. Before he told me the results, I would say, "Today's the day, my blood numbers are normal!" And he'd say in his low, monotone voice, "Not today." My response was always, "Tomorrow then."

While it was difficult to see the words clearly, I worked hard at reading my Bible and focused on verses that promised healing. Each day from what I read, the Lord impressed on my heart a particular Bible verse and it's meaning to me. I then wrote that verse on the ink board on the wall of my hospital room, where they accumulated one-by-one from the day I was admitted. I also listened to praise and worship music on my CD player each day. I thanked God for all the good things He had done for me and for His promises of healing, as I continued to look for and expect a miracle. I never even turned on the TV because I had more important things to do. Many of my friends brought me books, and I had time to actually read all of them.

I did my best to move around and stretch at least a few times per day. It was a bit difficult with an IV in my arm, but I managed. Taking a shower also had its challenges; I had to learn to function in the shower with my arm all wrapped up in cellophane in order to keep the water out of the IV connectors. To get there, I simply rolled the device that held the IV tubes and saline (or whatever medication they had prescribed for that day) into the bathroom and up to the shower entrance.

Once a day my room was thoroughly dusted and cleaned. I needed to wear a mask during the cleaning and for thirty minutes afterward so any dust would have time to settle. It was essential that the room stayed very clean because my condition left me highly susceptible to germs. In addition, all visitors to my room needed to wash their hands or put on gloves and keep a fair distance from me. Not only was it important to keep my room extremely free from germs, but the same was true of my food, which had to be specially prepared.

ACTS 3:16—IT'S FOR ME!

In the middle of the afternoon I was reading my Bible when my eyes crossed over the sixteenth verse in the third chapter of the Book of Acts. Those who have seen my Bible can attest to the fact that it looks like a rainbow from all the passages I have highlighted. But Acts 3:16? Not at all; it was simply black on white. Something amazing happened as I read those words: *On the basis of faith in His name, it is the name of Jesus which has strengthened this man whom you see and know; and the faith which comes through Him has given him this perfect health in the presence of you all* (Acts 3:16). I immediately received this verse in my heart as a personal promise and spoke out in a quiet voice, "That's going to be me. That's talking about me!" Instantly, I heard that still, small voice of the Lord say these incredible words to me: *That's the verse you're going to share with everyone on the day you're made whole.* Wow! It was so real. My eyes teared up with joy! Our God is an awesome God!

That's the verse you're going to share with everyone on the day you're made whole.

Treatment Begins

My first ATG transfusion began at 4:00 p.m. and lasted four hours. This specific battery of eight transfusions would be administered every twelve hours over the next four days, which meant I would be awakened at 4 a.m. for the next four days as well. That seemed to me an odd schedule, but what could I say? I was just the patient. I fell asleep early that evening but woke shortly after midnight with a nasty bout of hives. I had been warned about side effects and was experiencing a fairly bad reaction to the transfusion. They immediately administered an IV bag of Benadryl. Slowly the itching and swelling subsided, and I fell back to sleep for a few hours before they woke me for the next round. I geared myself up to remain faith-filled and positive over those next four days. I expected the ATG treatment to bring about the much-desired increase in my blood levels, thereby reducing my need to receive blood transfusions so frequently. There are risks to receiving any blood transfusion, but the risks increase with time and frequency.

The Nature of Transfusions

The doctors informed me that I would likely need ongoing blood transfusions after receiving the series of ATG transfusions, and after each transfusion, my hemoglobin and/or platelet levels would rise but then slowly decline over a period of days resulting in my need for another transfusion. The doctors pointed out that the human body often begins to reject transfused blood, and after two to three months of transfusions, my body could fail to respond to the new blood or it could reject it all together. This would bring on a new set of completely different life-threatening complications. Fewer transfusions are always best, but if I needed the blood, they had to give me the transfusions if it was still safe to do so.

The doctors were very careful not to give me more transfusions than I really needed, working to keep a balance between proper life support and over-transfusing in an effort to prevent my body from rejecting the donated blood.

THURSDAY, APRIL 12

A LETTER TO THE HOSPITAL STAFF

After the Lord spoke to me about how I would be sharing Acts 3:16 with everyone on the day I was made whole, I was unable to stop thinking about its significance. I got a sense from the Lord that I would be writing a letter of some kind to the hospital staff and that the Bible verses I added to the ink board in my room each day would be a part of the letter. It was impressed upon my heart that the letter would need to explain how I was miraculously healed, since the medical world would not be able to explain why or what happened once my tests were normal again. I sensed that I was supposed to prepare this letter immediately and that, when I was healed completely, I would deliver the letter, which I had already prepared during the time I was sick and still in the hospital. Initially, this seemed a bit far out, yet it was exactly in line with what I believed, so I acted on my belief and asked my wife to bring my laptop to the hospital. I told her that God was going to help me write a letter to the doctors and nurses who worked there and were caring for me.

DO THE DEEDS YOU DID AT FIRST

Later in the evening, as I was jumping about in the Scriptures, I came across Revelation Chapter 2. These passages *were* all highlighted in my Bible, and I was very familiar with them. This time, however, as I read them, I felt as if *my name* was being inserted into the verses. It became very personal. The chapter begins with a letter written to the church at Ephesus. As I read it, God spoke to my heart and told me to do more for Him by way of ministry—the kind of ministry I had done when I first became a believer in 1981. At that time, my heart was truly on fire for God. Jesus was the love of my life. It was a time when I continually shared my faith with others and told them of the goodness and love of God; God had used me on a regular basis to lead people into a personal relationship with their Creator. I was now reminded that I had *left my first love* and that Jesus wanted to be first in my life again, just like He was when

I first accepted Him into my life. He reminded me to *do the deeds I did at first.*

This was a special, personal moment with God; it was emotional, spiritual, and powerful all at the same time. I repented and asked forgiveness for my self-serving ways. I asked God to help me make the necessary changes in my life. He heard me, and He comforted me as I prayed. I drew strength from His Spirit and from His love. I believe He was calling me to share the wonderful message of His love with those I knew, those I would meet, and even those I didn't yet know. Not just now and then, or here and there, but in a more fervent and committed way. I still had time and work to do. Not only did I understand my responsibility, but I was now more certain than ever that God's hand was upon me and that I would be miraculously healed.

With this revelation, I prayed and told the Lord that as He opened doors for me, I would share His unconditional love with those who did not have a personal relationship with Him, as well as with those believers who might have lost their focus and closeness in their relationship with Him.

FRIDAY, APRIL 13

SURPRISE CALL FROM PASTOR HOLMES

I am not superstitious, so I treated Friday the 13th as just another day. However, that day would prove to be a far cry from just another day. About midday, I received a phone call from Pastor Holmes, the pastor who prayed for me two days prior to my being admitted to the hospital. From his car in Scottsdale, Arizona, he called my office and was transferred to my hospital room phone. We had not spoken since he had prayed for me, when we met at his church on Lake Street in Minneapolis. His message for me was profound. He told me the Lord had spoken to him and told him, *Jeff received a partial healing, and the rest of his healing will come if he is obedient to what you are to tell him.* I instantly realized that the partial healing was the recent stoppage of the internal bleeding that the doctors could not explain. It all began to make sense now; it was during Pastor Holmes' prayer—when I envisioned all those little white lights—that the *partial healing* had taken place! Right after that event my nose, face, and mouth had stopped bleeding.

Pastor Holmes had no idea I was in the hospital before making the call to me that day. He had no knowledge of the medical diagnosis. He only knew what the Lord had told him. Nearly in shock, I responded, "I'm all ears. What am I supposed to do?"

He humbly replied, "The Lord is asking you to sow into our new ministry here in Arizona—a ministry designed to get kids off the streets." He emphatically pointed out that he, himself, was not requesting any money but that the Lord was. He said I could send whatever—that it was totally up to me and if I only wanted to send five or ten dollars then do that. But he emphasized this: "Listen to what God tells you and send that amount."

When I initially heard this, I mentally backed off a bit but continued to listen. I knew for a fact that a miracle had already occurred, that my internal bleeding had stopped, and this provided instant credibility to what Pastor Holmes told me. I told him that I would speak with my wife, pray about it, and let him know tomorrow.

He said, "Fine. No problem." And we ended our phone call.

Being Obedient & Releasing the Money

When my wife arrived at the hospital later that evening, I shared with her what Pastor Holmes had told me. After discussing the specifics of all the interesting circumstances over the past eight days, we concluded that God was asking for our obedience with respect to helping this ministry in Arizona. Since we've always been givers, we looked forward to helping in this way. After agreeing on a respectable dollar amount, my wife planned to call Pastor Holmes first thing in the morning with the news. Her phone call set a series of events in motion—events that were, quite simply, beyond belief.

SATURDAY, APRIL 14
THE REST OF THE HEALING

Once each month, on a Saturday morning, I attended the 8:00 a.m. men's prayer breakfast held at Hosanna Church in Lakeville, Minnesota. Obviously, I was not in attendance on this particular Saturday. I later learned that around 9:00 a.m. the guys held a special prayer for me, knowing that I was recently admitted to the hospital and diagnosed with a serious disease. During their prayer for me, the Holy Spirit fell upon one of the attendees—Paul. The Lord spoke clearly and powerfully to Paul saying, *Paul, I want you to go to the hospital where Jeff Scislow is, pray for him, lay your left hand on his head, and tell him that he has been healed!* Immediately Paul's left arm heated up with a fire-like tingle, as if electricity were filling his arm! This incredible sensation was present from the tip of his fingers right up through his shoulder.

Now, Paul did not know me. He knew *of* me as a well-known Realtor, but he did not know me personally. He had no idea what hospital I was in or how to find me. He was a bit frightened but wanted to obey this direct command from the Lord. After lunch the condition of his arm had not changed. By 1:30 p.m., Paul decided to go back to church and look for a pastor. After combing the halls and offices, something prompted Paul to stick his head into the prayer chapel. He saw a familiar face and approached Greg, a man who had recently led a Bible study that Paul had attended. Feeling a sense of relief, Paul shared what had happened with Greg. As Paul was sharing this story with Greg, a smile appeared on Greg's face. When Paul finished speaking, Greg informed Paul that he worked at United Hospital and that Jeff was in room 4526. Paul was shocked!

It was clear that God had an assignment for Paul and was going to ensure it was completed.

At 7:30 p.m., Paul knocked on the door of my hospital room and slowly entered; humble and nervous, he told me this incredible story. He told me that his left arm was still hot and electrified. Tears of excitement and anticipation filled my eyes as I praised God for what was about to happen. Paul prayed, and when he placed his left hand on my head, I could feel the Holy Spirit—with fire and electricity—flow out of Paul's hand and into my body. I cried tears of joy that soon turned to uncontrolled laughter. It was truly incredible! It dawned on me that the rest of my healing had just occurred. God had moved powerfully in response to my obedience to His request that had come from Pastor Holmes' phone call. "It's happening just as God said it would," I expressed to Paul. "I've just been healed! Praise God! Hallelujah! This is so awesome!"

WRITE THE LETTER!

Later that evening, after Paul departed and just before I went to sleep, the Lord said to me, *Write the letter!* Filled with excitement over all that had happened, I quickly grabbed my laptop computer and began to write. I titled the letter, "I've Been Miraculously Healed" and dated it April 14, 2001. As I composed the letter, I eagerly anticipated how exciting it would be for me to deliver the letter and have all the doctors and nurses read it! I worked on it for a couple of hours.

I'VE BEEN MIRACULOUSLY HEALED!

On the basis of faith in His name, it is the name of Jesus which has strengthened this man whom you see and know; and the faith which comes through Him has given him (me) this perfect health in the presence of you all. (Acts 3:16)

I am writing this on Saturday April 14, 2001. As you know, I was admitted to my room 4526, United Hospital just one week ago today. I have been diagnosed as having no bone marrow (aplastic anemia), an extremely rare and deadly disease. I could not imagine how difficult this diagnosis would be for a patient that did not have a personal relationship & faith in Jesus Christ. My faith is enabling me to stand on God's promises as I believe for a full and complete healing, all in God's perfect timing. As each of you know, there is no fear residing in me.

The moment I arrived in my room I began adding Bible verses to the white ink board on the wall in my room for two reasons; one for my strength to endure this testing period and two, so that I could share them with you. Now that I have been in this room for one week, the Lord is telling me to write this very letter to you now, but not share it with you until my bone marrow and blood counts are once again normal. Due to the fact that you're now reading this, I have been undoubtedly and miraculously healed! Praise God!

I was blessed by each of you. Each doctor and each nurse who took care of me and tended to me shall not lose their reward for their kindness. God is faithful. Below are some of those verses that I have written on my wall, along with a few others. My prayer for each of you is that you come to know the Lord Jesus in an even more personal way. He loves you and He does perform on all His promises if we trust Him wholeheartedly! His Word is powerful & alive!

MY MIRACLE VERSES

Consider it all joy, my brethren when you encounter various trials, knowing that the testing of your faith produces endurance, and let endurance have its perfect result, that you may be perfect and complete, lacking in nothing.

(James 1:2-4)

Therefore humble yourselves under the mighty hand of God, that He may exalt you at the proper time, casting all your anxiety upon Him, because He cares for you ... After you have suffered a little while, the God of all grace, who called you to His eternal glory in Christ, will Himself perfect, confirm, strengthen and establish you.

(1 Peter 5:6-7,10)

For the Word of God is living and active and sharper than any two-edged sword, and piercing as far as the division of soul and spirit, of both joints and marrow, and able to judge the thoughts and intentions of the heart.

(Hebrews 4:12)

No weapon formed against you [me] shall prosper.

(Isaiah 54:17)

The angel of the Lord encamps around those who fear Him, and rescues them.

(Psalm 34:7)

The righteous cry, and the Lord hears and delivers them out of all their troubles.

(Psalm 34:17)

Many are the afflictions of the righteous; but the Lord delivers him out of them all.

(Psalm 34:19)

For I know the plans that I have for you, declares the Lord, plans for welfare and not for calamity, to give you a future and a hope.

(Jeremiah 29:11)

My son, give attention to My words; incline your ear to My sayings; do not let them depart from your sight; keep them in the midst of your heart. For they are life to those who find them and health to all their whole body.

(Proverbs 4:20-22)

Beloved, do not be surprised at the fiery ordeal among you, which comes upon you for your testing, as though some strange thing were happening to you; but to the degree you share in the sufferings of Christ, keep on rejoicing, so that also at the revelation of His glory, you may rejoice with exultation.

(1 Peter 4:12-13)

Therefore I say to you, all things for which you pray and ask, believe that you have received them, and they will be granted you.

(Mark 11:24)

Whatever you ask in My name, that will I do, so that the Father may be glorified in the Son. If you ask Me anything in My name, I will do it.

(John 14:13-14)

If you abide in Me, and My words abide in you, ask whatever you wish, and it will be done for you.

(John 15:7)

For we walk by faith, not by sight.

(2 Corinthians 5:7)

For God has not given us the spirit of fear; but of power, and of love, and of a sound mind.

(2 Timothy 1:7)

Therefore, do not throw away your confidence, which has a great reward. For you have need of endurance, so that when you have done the will of God, you may receive what was promised.

(Hebrews 10:35-36)

FORMER PATIENT,
JEFF SCISLOW

SUNDAY, APRIL 15
EASTER SUNDAY

After the amazing day I just had, I could not wait for the doctor to roll in mid-morning and deliver me the miraculous results of my 6:30 a.m. blood draw. I felt especially honored to be able to experience my miracle on Easter Sunday. I was so filled with anticipation that I began buzzing the nurse on the call button and asking when the doctor would arrive. The doctor finally arrived, but the miracle had not. In fact, my blood levels had dropped considerably from the day before. Multiple transfusions were ordered, both platelets and hemoglobin. For most of the day, as I received bag after bag of blood, I thought to myself, *What happened?* I played the events of the last few days over and over in my mind. They were so closely knit together, yet each seemed miraculous on their own. Paul was given a clear message for me, "Jeff, you are healed!" I could not figure that part out. I had expected to be healed, but I was still very sick, lying there in bed with all kinds of needles in me as I received multiple blood transfusions.

During the course of this long day, I was reminded of 1 Peter 5:6: *Therefore, humble yourselves under the mighty hand of God, that He may exalt you at the proper time.* I realized that I needed to be patient and continue trusting God, especially for His timing on the healing I was expecting. I continued to optimistically believe that my miracle would arrive, if not on this day then the next!

MONDAY, APRIL 16

Filled once again with the anticipation of receiving my miraculous healing, I looked forward to the doctor's visit and the report from the day's blood draw. To my disappointment, there was no indication of a *healing*. The blood numbers were only slightly higher, even after receiving all the blood transfusions the day before.

TAKE YOUR THOUGHTS CAPTIVE

I started to feel like I was fighting a losing battle and that maybe the doctors were right. Fear was knocking on my emotional door, and I was slipping into what I call "no man's land," which is not the place anyone wants to be. After experiencing these thoughts for a few minutes, I caught myself from falling deeper into the trap of negativity and fear. I needed to stay positive and take those thoughts *captive to the obedience of Christ* (2 Corinthians 10:5). Each time I had a fearful, anxious, or doubting thought, I made a conscious effort to capture and resist it. I would counter-punch such thoughts with Bible verses that promised something positive, often speaking the verses out loud. I sought to make a regular, determined effort to do this—to capture any negative thinking and to do it each and every day, for as many days as it took, until the victory was mine.

Taking thoughts captive is a learned behavior fueled by faith. As I continued to practice this, I gained strength each and every time. As I resisted the devil (his lies and the negative thoughts he initiated), he fled from me, and in the midst of these emotional and spiritual battles, I regularly spoke these words out loud: *The Lord has not given me a spirit of fear, but of love, power and a sound mind* (2 Timothy 1:7).

TUESDAY, APRIL 17

DANIEL PERSISTED FOR TWENTY-ONE DAYS!

After providing my seventy-fifth tube of blood since March, I popped in a cassette my friend had delivered to me the night before. In the message on the cassette, Pastor Chip Brim gave a sermon about the significance of Daniel 10 and how it relates to prayer being answered. I carefully read Daniel 10 over and over again and learned that Daniel prayed to God for a revelation but did not get an answer to his prayer for twenty-one days. Daniel's prayer was heard on the first day, but Daniel did not receive the response until the twenty-first day. Immediately after Daniel began to pray, the answer to his prayer was sent from heaven with the Angel of the Lord; however, before the answer could be delivered, demonic forces in the heavenly realm opposed the delivery of the answered prayer and battled to keep the answer from him.

As the battle between angelic and demonic forces waged on, Daniel persisted in prayer and fasting, making a clear choice not to give up. On the twenty-first day of Daniel's persistent prayer, the archangel Michael was dispatched from heaven to fight alongside the Angel of the Lord. They overpowered the demonic forces, allowing Daniel to receive the answer to his prayer! This is a wonderful image of spiritual warfare and the subsequent spiritual breakthrough that awaits those who do not give up.

THE GOAL LINE DEFENSE

In his sermon, Brim, a former football coach, described a vision that the Lord had given him years before. In the vision, the Lord took Brim to a very interesting football game during which he was neither on the field nor in the bleachers; rather, he was hovering above the field with a clear view of everything. From this vantage point, the Lord illustrated to Brim what he already knew from his own experience: *It is much easier to move the football from your own end of the field or even from mid-field, but as you enter your opponent's end of the field, it becomes more difficult to move the ball. In fact, when you get down to the one-yard line, the defense puts in its biggest and toughest players to prevent you from scoring a touchdown.*

The same is true in the spiritual world, the Lord told Brim. *When people in need are on the cusp of receiving their miracle, their healing, their answered prayer, the enemy (Satan) will put in his best defensive players to prevent a touchdown. He will dispatch his evil, demonic warriors to instill doubt, fear, uncertainty, and chaos to get them to give up, cave in, quit, and throw in the towel; and if they do, they lose, and the enemy wins. However, if one perseveres like Daniel, the touchdown* **will** *be scored, the miracle* **will** *arrive, and the faithful recipient* **will** *tell the world what Jesus has done! That is the last thing Satan wants, so he will put up a hell of a fight.*

In the vision, the Lord then revealed to Brim millions and millions of people, young and old, who had died on the one-yard line. They never made it across. They got close, but they never got over the goal line. They never scored their touchdown, never received their healing, and never got their miracle. When the enemy challenged their emotions and faith with all his weapons, he overcame them.

Wow, I thought, *This is really heavy!* I gained much strength from both Brim's message and Daniel 10. I was determined not to be a casualty on the one-yard line; my faith would not fail! I would trust God completely, would not waver, and would expect a miracle no matter how long this journey took! I was drawn to the verses that say; *My righteous one shall live by faith; and if he shrinks back, My soul has no pleasure in him. But we are not of those who shrink back to destruction, but of those who have faith to the preserving of the soul* (Hebrews 10:38-39).

BATTLES IN LIFE ARE SPIRITUAL IN NATURE

Ephesians 6:12 reads; *For our struggle is not against flesh and blood, but against the rulers, against the powers, against the world forces of this darkness, against the spiritual forces of wickedness in the heavenly places.* This is exactly what Daniel experienced; a spiritual battle. Daniel did not give up and neither would I! I needed to be patient and believe God for His perfect timing. Hebrews 6:11-12 says to *show the same diligence so as to realize the full assurance of hope until the end, so that you may not be sluggish, but imitators of those who through faith and patience inherit the promises.* And Hebrews 10:35-36 reads; *Therefore, do not throw away your confidence, which has a great reward. For you have need for endurance, so that when you have done the will of God, you may receive what was promised.*

WEDNESDAY, APRIL 18
I AM HEALED!

My mind continually replayed the events that had occurred since I had arrived at the hospital. I repeatedly went over the details in an attempt to gain a better understanding of what was happening to me and what I needed to do next. I was particularly intrigued and perplexed by what Paul had told me the prior Saturday night. The Lord told Paul, *Pray for Jeff. Lay your left hand on his head and tell him he has been healed.*

Maybe Paul got it wrong, I thought. *Did he say it correctly? Maybe he was supposed to say, Jeff, you **will** be healed.*

But I had to believe that what Paul said was exactly what he was supposed to say. What was the significance of telling me I had been healed when in fact I was not yet healed? I was still without bone marrow, without an immune system, and susceptible to dying at any time! Then, finally, it dawned on me! It was as if the Lord downloaded a profound answer to the perplexing question I had been trying to solve. The Lord's message to me was very simple: *Jeff, you have been healed.* Paul was instructed to *tell Jeff he has been healed.* The past tense of this message was powerful! I was *already* healed!

Immediately, I thought of a familiar verse, which states, *by His wounds you were healed* (1 Peter 2:24). By Jesus' wounds or stripes (from flogging, beating, and crucifixion), we *are* healed. His sacrifice on the cross paid the price for my healing. Jesus did not *just* die for my sins but also for my sicknesses! I turned to Isaiah 53:5 and learned from this verse that Jesus died on the cross for three things: my sins, my sicknesses, and my well-being.

I now had a greater sense of God's goodness. He had sent other obedient believers to deliver several messages to me in order to facilitate my understanding of something incredibly powerful. And the faith I had up to this point just rose to new heights. I came to realize that I had already been healed in the spiritual sense. As a result of God's Word, the sacrifice Jesus made when He died on the cross, and my own solid faith, I had already been healed! It is a promise!

Furthermore, I realized I was in a spiritual battle, positioned on the one-yard line, attempting to score a touchdown. Through faith and persistence I knew I would cross the goal line, score the touchdown, and receive *physical* healing! If I maintained this belief and did not give up, I knew I would win the battle. As I intensely and diligently sought an answer of the meaning *Tell Jeff he has been healed*, I was rewarded with a revelation of great intensity and meaning!

SATURDAY, APRIL 21

Nothing of significance occurred for a few days, and I followed my personal routine religiously. Each day I had blood drawn, listened to praise music, read the Bible, posted one verse on my ink board, read from a book or two, and worked on my thoughts. I wanted to ensure each and every thought was aligned with the expectation of what I was telling everyone I believed. I found this to be extremely important for my own well-being. Whatever promise

I found in the Bible, which applied to my situation or my need, I stood on without wavering.

THE PRAYER OF JABEZ

I began sensing that the Lord wanted to work on my heart and reveal things that would help me endure and better understand my current journey. A few days earlier, one of my visitors had brought me *The Prayer of Jabez*. I had initially placed it on the ledge along the wall in my room, but tonight I decided to pick it up and read it. I was able to finish the book before going to bed that night and prayed Jabez's prayer out loud. I prayed it intensely just as I imagined Jabez himself must have prayed it, expecting to receive the very things for which I petitioned; *Oh that You would bless me indeed and enlarge my border, and that Your hand might be with me, that You would keep me from harm that it may not pain me! And God granted him what he requested* (1 Chronicles 4:10).

SUNDAY, APRIL 22

HINDERED PRAYER?

The day after diligently praying the Jabez prayer, I experienced some interesting things that kept me focused on my anticipated miracle of healing. I felt drawn to read a passage from 1 Corinthians 11:30-31; *For this reason many among you are weak and sick, and a number sleep* [have died]. *But if we judged ourselves rightly, we would not be judged.* I knew that prayer could be hindered, and since I obviously did not want mine to be hindered, I set out to examine myself and ask God to reveal anything He wanted me to work on. He showed me several important things about myself.

HONOR YOUR WIFE

The first area that the Lord directed my attention was the relationship between my wife and my parents and how I had been dealing with the challenges between them. For over fourteen years I tried to bridge the gap between them during times of disagreement and misunderstanding. In each instance I played the peacemaker, trying to mediate or negotiate, and this had been causing friction between my wife and me for years. That afternoon, during a phone call with my wife, the topic strayed to disharmonious family matters. However, this time, instead of automatically shifting into peacemaker mode, I felt compelled to listen. After listening at length to my wife, the familiar stories that I had heard many times before took on a new and different meaning. The way I processed the same information was different too—so different that it brought tears to my eyes. I realized that day, by divine revelation, that my wife simply wanted me to defend her position—to take her side. As we talked, my tears turned to laughter; the joy of the Lord was upon me, and a fresh internal healing occurred both in my wife and me.

Later, I spoke with my parents about what had transpired. I expressed to my parents that I loved them very much and respected their position as well but that my true role was that of my wife's defender. Although it must have been surprising after so many years, they handled it very well. They understood and respected what I had to say. Before going to bed, I recalled my prayer the night before: *Lord, bless me INDEED!* And, indeed, that is what He did. In the course of a few hours, I experienced a breakthrough for a problem that had gone on for fourteen years.

TUESDAY, APRIL 24

The ninety-fifth tube of blood taken from my body showed that my blood counts were still at dangerously low levels with no sign that the ATG treatment was having any success. A platelet transfusion was ordered for me later that morning. Still, although the medical professionals continued to say I was *really, really sick,* I felt stronger all the time—not necessarily in a physical sense, but mentally, emotionally, and spiritually.

HOW'S BUSINESS?

Since my arrival at the hospital, the springtime real estate market in the Twin Cities had been quite robust. I was mindful that I had a commissioned position and needed to do whatever I could to continue receiving an income, as my insurance did not cover loss of commissions. While in the confines of my hospital room, I took calls from existing clients who had questions regarding the marketing of their home. When prospects or clients called in and asked for me, my wife or staff would reply that I was in the hospital for a few days for observation with low white blood cell counts but fine otherwise and still able to take calls. By using conference calls, I was able to negotiate offers over the phone with my clients and go through the process of listing homes.

The business was blessed—certainly more than the previous fall! We continued to tell our clients and prospects that I was simply being held for observation for a few more days. From a disadvantaged position, our new system had produced four listings and four sales in April.

THURSDAY, APRIL 26

The morning blood draw revealed another extremely low platelet count, and it had become apparent that the platelet transfusions were not increasing the levels like they once had. On top of this, the platelet levels were dropping more rapidly after each transfusion. This was clearly not a good sign, but I refused to worry. I kept thanking the Lord for all the good things that were happening. I stood on His Word and stayed the course of expecting a miracle!

In the middle of the morning I was informed that I would be moved to a new room. I did not want to move, because I simply felt comfortable in my room where I had been for nineteen days. To my delight, however, the new room had a real sense of life and positive energy in it—something rare for a room in an oncology ward. It offered a much better layout than the room I had been in, was larger, and even had a better view. I realized that something as simple as a little hospital room could mean so much when surrounded by unfortunate circumstances such as mine.

FRIDAY, APRIL 27

Day after day I sought guidance from the Lord to help me understand if there was anything else standing in the way of my healing. If a hindrance existed, I wanted it identified so I could do whatever it took to remove it.

HUMBLE YOURSELF

Just after 11:00 p.m. I finished listening to a wonderful tape series by my friend, Pastor Joe Braucht. The tapes, entitled *Renewing a Right Heart,* discussed the importance of being right with God and the steps we can take to get into a right relationship with Him. This is exactly what I sought—a deeper walk with Him in all areas of my life. As a result of listening to the tapes and contemplating the message, the Lord revealed something to me: I heard a still, small voice say, *Why do you think of yourself as more important than others?* I was puzzled at first but then experienced many insightful thoughts and emotions about how I truly viewed myself. For years, others had praised me for my successes. I had grown proud of my accomplishments. I compared myself with others—consciously as well as unconsciously. Even though I aimed for humility, pride had a way of sneaking up on me.

The Lord was very kind and gentle as He asked me again, *Why do you think of yourself as more important than others?* I had no answer other than, "I am sorry." I was overcome with emotion and cried, feeling saddened by my past actions. I buried my head in my pillow and cried for thirty minutes. Then, a sense of relief and joy fell over me, and I began laughing out loud. Once again, the joy of the Lord came as a confirmation of a good work completed within me.

As I examined my heart, the Lord revealed pieces of my life that He wanted to see me improve. I did not want to end up like the Corinthians to whom Paul spoke—the weak, sick, or those that had died. I wanted healing to manifest in my life, and I was willing to do whatever I needed to do.

LOVE

More verses from God's Word came to me to strengthen me as I examined myself. In Luke 10:27-28, Jesus says, *You shall love the Lord your God with all your heart, and with all your soul, and with all your strength, and with all your mind; and love your neighbor as yourself . . . Do this and you will live.* In 1 Corinthians 13:1-3, Paul writes, *If I speak with the tongues of men and of angels, but do not have LOVE, I have become a noisy gong or a clanging cymbal. If I have the gift of prophecy, and know all mysteries and all knowledge; and if I have all faith, so as to remove mountains, but do not have LOVE, I am nothing. And if I give all my possessions to feed the poor, and if I surrender my body to be burned, but do not have LOVE, it profits me NOTHING!*

After reading these verses, I thought about how busy society had become, how the *love* of so many had grown cold, and how everyone seemed to be so self-absorbed. I continued to examine myself in light of these verses, and I turned to this Biblical description of society in the days preceding the return of Jesus Christ: *But realize this, that in the last days difficult times will come. For men will be lovers of self, lovers of money, boastful, arrogant, revilers, disobedient to parents, ungrateful, unholy, unloving, irreconcilable, malicious gossips, without self-control, brutal, haters of good, treacherous, reckless, conceited, lovers of pleasure rather than lovers of God; holding to a form of godliness, although they have denied its power; avoid such men as these . . . always learning and never able to come to the knowledge of the truth* (2 Timothy 3:1-7).

Tuesday, May 1

Platelets Nosedive

My morning blood draw revealed my lowest platelet count since arriving at the hospital. I fought discouragement, as it was clear that my ATG treatment had failed. The specialists at the University of Minnesota, along with the oncologists at United Hospital, had all agreed that if the treatment were to work we would see results within two weeks. Two weeks had passed, and my condition had only worsened.

A White Halo of Light

Later in the morning, Erin, the young woman who regularly cleaned my room, was going about her cleaning responsibilities as she and I talked. I often shared with her the many things I had experienced while staying in the hospital, along with my full expectation of a complete healing. While we were talking, she suddenly stopped and stared for a moment, as if she was assessing something. She began to describe a vision of what she was seeing in the room: *I see a circular aura, like a halo over your head, and a white beam of light ascending up into the sky.* I asked her where the beam of light went and she replied, *To the throne of God.*

Upon hearing this, all discouragement from my low platelet count disappeared. I did not know what this meant, nor did I try to figure it out. I was simply amazed once again at how I continued to receive messages, visitors, tapes, visions, and revelations from God just when I needed them most, and this day was no exception!

THE SEARCH FOR MARROW DONOR

When it became evident that the ATG treatment had failed to produce results, the doctors knew it was time to proceed to option two—a possible bone marrow transplant. They conducted a search on the worldwide database to locate a matching marrow donor for me. No match was found so they requested that my three siblings, Jyl, Jim, and Ed, be tested as a hopeful match.

Even with a perfect marrow match, because of my age, there was only a slight chance of successfully surviving the transplant procedure. If I survived the procedure and the marrow was not rejected immediately, I was told I might have two years before I would become susceptible to bone marrow rejection or relapse. The odds were slim to none that I would live very long, if at all, and, as strange as it may sound, I had been so blessed during the preceding few weeks that I felt like the luckiest person on earth. I had seen the Lord there for me every time I was in need—whether it was a physical, emotional, or spiritual need. God had been there right on schedule. It was truly amazing! So I continued to wait on the Lord without any fear. I read from Isaiah 40:31; *Yet those who wait on the Lord will gain new strength; they will mount up with wings like eagles, they will run and not get tired, they will walk and not become weary.*

BLOOD TEST RESULTS WHILE IN THE HOSPITAL

Actual CBC (complete blood count) test results reveal dangerously low levels during my 28 days in the hospital.

980-12444

UNITED HOSPITAL
St. Paul, Minnesota

PROTOCOL NUMBER: _____

DIAGNOSIS: _____

DATE:	4-8	4-8	4-9	4-10	4-11	4-12	4-13	4-14	4/15	4/17	4/18	4/19	4/20	4/21	4/2
HEMATOLOGY															
HGB (F:12-16, M:14-18)	5.9	8.5	8.0		9.5	9.6	8.7	8.4	8.0	11.1	11.3	9.9	11.1	10.7	10.
WBC (4.8-10.8)	700	400	400		500	500	200	300	300	400	500	500	700	900	6L
Polys															
Bands															
Lymphs															
Monos															
Periph Blasts															
Platelets (150,000 — / 300,000)	2,000	26,000	22,000		12,000	7,000	23,000	11,000	9,000	40,000		9,000	14,000	9,000	23
Protime (11-13)															
PTT (24-36)															
Thrombin Time (8-14)															
FSP (< 10)															
Fibrinogen (200-600)															
BLOOD PRODUCTS REQUIRED	150 PLT	3units PRBC													

DATE:	4/23	4/24	4/25	4/26	4/27	4-28	4-29	4-30	5/1	5/2	5/3	5/4			
HEMATOLOGY															
HGB (F:12-16, M:14-18)	9.9	9.3	9.2	8.7	7.6	9.5	9.5	9.1	9.0	8.9	8.5	10.6			
WBC (4.8-10.8)	900	900	900	1100	800	1.1	1.5	1.3	1.3	1.1	1.0	1.3			
Polys															
Bands															
Lymphs															
Monos															
Periph Blasts															
Platelets (150,000 — / 300,000)	10K	36K	14K	7K	26K	20K	4K	12K	5,000	43K	32K	24K			
Protime (11-13)															
PTT (24-36)															
Thrombin Time (8-14)															
FSP (< 10)															
Fibrinogen (200-600)															
BLOOD PRODUCTS REQUIRED															
BONE MARROW BIOPSY Blasts															
Specify Protocol and agents.															

HEMATOLOGY ONCOLOGY

WEDNESDAY, MAY 3

They drew my one hundred and fifteenth tube of blood as the team of doctors continued to monitor the ravaging effects of the aplastic anemia. The test results revealed a continued drop in my hemoglobin level, and a double-bag transfusion of red cells was ordered.

GOD CONSIDERS ME UNIQUE

The oncologist stopped by my room later than normal that day with the results of my siblings' bone marrow tests. There was no match, and, somehow expecting this, I quickly responded by saying, "Amen! God considers me unique! He is just making it clear to everyone that it will be Him, and Him alone, that will heal me." The doctor just stared at me in silence for a moment before informing me that I was going home the next day because there was nothing else they could do. Hearing this, I began to believe I would be healed miraculously by morning so all the doctors and nurses could witness it. I thought to myself this was God's perfect timing, and felt tomorrow would be the day!

THURSDAY, MAY 4

The oncologist arrived with the test results from my morning blood draw. There was no change in my condition; I was still without bone marrow, and my blood numbers had declined again. The platelets had fallen to the point where I required another transfusion. The oncologist planned to meet with me after the transfusion in order to give me crucial instructions in my fight for survival.

A MINI PROGNOSIS

The afternoon had arrived, the platelets had been transfused, and I was about to be discharged from the security of the oncology ward at United Hospital. Before leaving, I met with the nurse before seeing the oncologist. She gave me three informational, preprinted pages on *How to Deal with Low Red Blood Cells*, *How to Deal with Low White Blood Cells*, and *How to Deal with Low Platelets*. It is interesting to note that my sheets had been edited—they crossed out the part where it stated that my counts would get better. Their message was clear: *I was not going to get better.*

I refused to let this bother me. God had a plan and a promise for me—a plan for me to be healed completely from this affliction.

THE DOCTOR'S PARTING WORDS

When I met with the oncologist, he related the following message: "Keep an eye on your temperature. Should you develop a fever of 101 degrees, get back in here right away. If you experience any pain, rashes, or uncontrolled bleeding, get back here as quickly as possible. You will need blood transfusions every three to four days so set up a regular schedule with the front desk. We will continue to look for a marrow match for you and will let you know if we locate a donor. But for now, stay away from your kids, don't kiss your wife, get rid of your pets, and don't go out in public unless you absolutely have to. And if you do, wear a mask."

With these parting words, I walked out of the fortress I had called home for the past twenty-eight days into a world filled with germs. I knew I had to be extremely careful or I could die from a common cold. I was determined to do all I could to bring about the expected miracle. I reminded myself that I was healed no matter what I encountered. No matter what others said, I was going to stand firm on God's promises. I was going to cross the goal line and score my touchdown. The victory was mine if I didn't lose heart and give up!

Stay away from your kids, don't kiss your wife, get rid of your pets, and don't go out in public unless you absolutely have to; and if you do, wear a mask.

CHAPTER 4

— SENT HOME WITHOUT HOPE —

*. . . do not throw away your confidence, which has a great
reward. For you have need of endurance, so that when you have
done the will of God, you may receive what was promised.*
—HEBREWS 10:35–36

CHAPTER 4

The oncologist sent me home from the hospital with little to no hope for survival. I was provided a long list of cautions and conditions designed to keep me free from germs while the doctors searched for a matching marrow donor. A secluded living space was set up for me in the basement of my home, and it was off limits to the children and our pets. My wife brought me meals, and at times I went upstairs to eat when the children were not immediately present.

After a few days at home, I decided to send a brief email to a dozen or so acquaintances. I simply asked for their prayers—I did not want to reveal too much information about my personal battle with this disease and wanted this part of my life to remain private. Immediately after I sent that first brief email, however, the Lord told me to open up, be transparent, and share with *everyone* what was happening in my life and how I trusted Him to heal me. I wrestled with this and came up with an excuse, saying, "I know You are going to heal me, but just in case You don't I do not want to be a stumbling block to all those people and cause them to lose faith in You."

I did not hear anything from the Lord. It's as if He folded His arms and turned His back to me. A few days passed and still nothing. I thought deeply; then it dawned on me: I was making a big mistake, two of them! First, I was certainly not acting in faith when I said to God, "But just in case You don't heal me . . ." And second, God asked me to do something, and I was refusing. I immediately asked God to forgive me for such foolishness on my part, and in a revering way I said, "God, You don't need me to watch Your back, but if You don't heal me it won't be my problem—I am going to tell everyone everything."

Instantly, as if God was waiting for me to say those words, He spoke to my heart saying, *I am going to show Myself strong through you, before the eyes of many people.* I was in complete awe! This was another promise from God that He was going to heal me but also that He had some sort of plan to use me as I tell everyone everything. At that moment of joy, excitement, and humility, I began gathering thoughts as to what I needed to share with everyone.

I am going to show Myself strong through you, before the eyes of many people.

Within a few days, I began to compose a second email. This lengthy, multi-page email went into great detail with respect to what had transpired over the past year—from the Seattle-based dot-com experience to my twenty-eight day stay in the hospital. After several days of writing this email, it was sent to over 22,000 recipients! I had a large database of friends and real estate agents from around the country, and I made sure they each heard from me. I needed to bring *everyone* up to speed on what had occurred in my life over the past year in order to set the stage for all to witness my expected miracle.

Little did I know at the time, but those emails would become the pages you are now reading. Basically, what you have read to this point has been content from what was contained in that second email. The pages that follow are actual parts of a third, and subsequent, emails that I sent from the basement of my home, after I was sent home from the hospital and as I continued on my "journey to a miracle." (The content of the emails has been slightly edited for readability, but, beyond this simple editing, it is virtually presented word-for-word.)

MAY 19, 2001

To this point in my journey I continued to be utterly amazed at how all the events and details were so positively interwoven. Experiencing these increased my faith to new levels. I absolutely believed that a miracle was forthcoming; I had total faith in this, even though medical evidence pointed to something completely different.

WALKING BY FAITH, NOT BY SIGHT

As I listened to all the reports, opinions, and advice from the medical world, it was quite clear that the odds were greatly against surviving. I believed all the details provided to me thus far by the doctors were sound. They provided me with an accurate medical analysis. Was it good news? No way. It really stunk. The diagnosis and prognosis were reality, and I could not go into denial; I had to deal with the circumstances at hand. All the findings and analysis came from the world we know and understand as the *sight* realm, but there is another realm out there called the *faith* realm.

According to 2 Corinthians 5:7, Christians are to *walk by faith, and not by sight*. We are to trust in what God says in His Word, even if it seems to go against what appears to be reality. I believe God, especially when His Word says; *without faith it is impossible to please Him, for he who comes to God must believe that He is, and that He is a rewarder of those who diligently seek Him* (Hebrews 11:6).

Nothing is impossible with God. Just look at what has already happened; I could not be any more blessed! In fact, I felt like the most blessed person in the world because I knew I was going to experience a miracle that not everyone gets to experience. God said He was going to show Himself strong through me so why should I have any doubts? And He said it would happen before the eyes of many people!

JUST HOW MANY PEOPLE DID JESUS HEAL?

Time and time again, Scripture tells us that Jesus healed *all* that were brought to Him. And John 1:1,14 says; *In the beginning was the Word, and the Word was with God, and the Word was God. And the Word became flesh, and dwelt among us.* In the book of Matthew we see that Jesus is the living Word of God. He is the Word. Jesus healed with His Word (Matthew 8:16). *He sent His Word and healed them, and delivered them from their destructions* (Psalm 107:20). *Jesus Christ is the same yesterday and today and forever* (Hebrews

13:8), and God says in Malachi 3:6; *I, the Lord, do not change.* So you can see, Jesus is the Word, and He healed all who were afflicted with sickness. He does not need to be physically present to heal, because physical healing is as available today as it was 2,000 years ago!

Verses with Big Promises

One of the simplest verses that I clung to while in the hospital was John 15:7: *If you abide in Me, and My words abide in you, ask whatever you wish, and it will be done for you.* This is pretty direct with no gray area. *Abide* means to trust, to follow, to lean on, to latch onto, and to obey. *If* I do this, *then* God says He will grant any request I bring before Him. Likewise, from 1 John 3:22, we see that *if* we do our part, *then* God will do His part: *and whatever we ask we receive from Him, because we keep His commandments and do the things that are pleasing in His sight.*

Another terrific passage that ends in a promise, providing you do your part, is: *Ask, and it will be given to you; seek, and you will find; knock, and it will be opened to you. For everyone who asks receives, and he who seeks finds, and to him who knocks it will be opened. Or what man is there among you who, when his son asks for a loaf, will give him a stone? Or if he asks for a fish, he will not give him a snake, will he? If you then, being evil, know how to give good gifts to your children, how much more will your Father who is in heaven give what is good to those who ask Him!* (Matthew 7:7-11).

His Promise

God is faithful to His Word. I knew the miracle would not arrive because of me nor because I was a special favorite of God but because God is able and willing to do it for His glory. He loves me, and because He has already promised to do so in His Word, I was simply standing firm on His promise!

Stay Away from Crowds

When I left the hospital with a dangerously low white blood cell count, I was told to stay away from crowds because of all the germs, etc. My plan was to spend most of my time in my basement.

The third day out of the hospital, however, I felt compelled to go to a local Sunday evening church service to hear a minister from Indiana by the name of Steve Munsey. I did not know who he was. I had never heard him speak. I just felt I needed to go.

This was the first time I ventured out of my house to be around a crowd so it was necessary for me to wear my surgical mask to fend off airborne germs—I must admit this was a humbling experience. Not only did Pastor Munsey deliver an incredible message that night, he said something profound—something that appeared to come out of nowhere. In the middle of his powerful and animated delivery—and believe me he was on a roll—he suddenly froze in his tracks for a few seconds as if he was listening to something. The room was dead silent, and then he said this: *The Lord is telling me that there is someone here tonight whom the doctors have told does not have long to live. But God is going to remove that sickness that has come against you and add fifteen years to your life.*

"The Lord is telling me that there is someone here tonight who the doctors have told does not have long to live. But God is going to remove that sickness that has come against you and add fifteen years to your life."

All along, God has provided little signs, words, or messages to help me, to keep me strong, and to perfect my faith. By faith, I chose to take ownership of that prophetic Word—it *was* meant for me! Until that night, I had no desire to leave the confines of my home. I believe that the Lord not only wanted me to hear the general message, but He also wanted to deliver me a personal one through Pastor Munsey.

GETTING AN UNEASY FEELING

After a couple days of being out of the hospital and living (basically) out of my basement, I began getting an uneasy feeling about a powerful drug the doctors had recently prescribed for me. The drug, called Cyclosporine, is a preparatory drug used on patients who may undergo a bone marrow transplant, as it further suppresses any immune activity. Since I had virtually no immune system, I was not really sure why I was on this drug in the first place. I simply went along with the doctor's recommendation. I began to sense that this was the wrong thing to be doing. I had always taken every pill or medication the doctors prescribed, but this time something was different.

ONE OF MY TENANTS STOPS BY

On May 5, I had a brief business conversation on the phone with Monique, a tenant at one of my rental properties. During our talk, I mentioned the diagnosis I had received from the doctors. Two days later, Monique showed up at my home. She told me that for the past two days she had been praying about whether or not to bring some *interesting material* over to me. She went on to tell me she had not been getting an answer to her prayer, but while driving in her car, she began praying again. As she pulled up to the next intersection, the car immediately in front of her had a bumper sticker with one word on it: YES! That was the answer to her prayer, and she immediately drove to my home!

The *interesting material* that Monique shared was a book and VHS tape on herbs and natural healing by Dr. Richard Schulze. She and her husband Tom had been given this information by someone at their church and began using the products a year earlier. They testified to the health benefits they'd received as a result of taking the products, and the material revealed how these natural herbs had healed over 10,000 of this particular herbal doctor's patients! These patients had cancer, AIDS, heart conditions, tumors, Alzheimer's, blood disorders, and numerous other diseases. It was quite intriguing to read through the medical information that was presented along with the numerous testimonials.

As I continued to comb through the information on natural healing, I kept in mind the circumstances under which I had received this information—yet another believer who prayed for direction and was led to deliver this information into my hands. My wife and I began talking about the Cyclosporine. She too had developed an uneasy feeling about my taking it. We could not quite pin it down, however. Nevertheless, I made the decision to cut my daily dosage from 800 mg to 600 mg without discussing it with my oncologist.

OFF THE MEDS

On the morning of May 10, I began doing additional research on the use of Cyclosporine and numerous warnings and side effects (renal dysfunction, structural kidney damage, nephrotoxicity, hepatotoxicity, high blood pressure, neoplasms such as lymphoma and carcinomas of the skin, and several others). Midday, I made the choice to stop taking Cyclosporine altogether.

Emotionally, stopping the medication caused me to feel as though I had lost a lifeline. While taking the meds, I was able to maintain hope that something positive would result, such as a return to the health condition I so desperately desired. But now that I had chosen to stop taking them, the hopeful lifeline had been cut. It was just one of those little emotions that I needed to work through.

SIDE EFFECTS

Later in the day on May 10, while at the doctor's office to receive a platelet transfusion, I had my blood pressure tested—it was quite high, and the next day I began noticing an intense dull pain in my kidneys. I realized I was most likely experiencing the side effects of Cyclosporine and began to understand why I had been getting that funny feeling about the drug. I thanked the Lord for prompting that feeling, and within a week after I stopped taking the Cyclosporine, my kidney pain went away, a rash that had begun developing had almost disappeared, and my blood pressure dropped steadily back to normal after peaking at 186/126.

HERBAL PROGRAM BEGINS

On the afternoon of May 11, I finally came to the decision to begin the herbal program which would cleanse my body and build it up with natural herbs. This is what my heart was telling me to do. The products included a Superfood breakfast mix of herbs, vitamins and minerals, and a product designed to ensure several bowel movements daily.

TILL THE SOIL

Even though I felt that the Lord had paved the way for me to get off medication and begin an herbal program, I was still praying for a confirmation that I was making the right choice. The warnings and risks from the medical world with respect to taking herbs with my condition seemed very real, and I was certainly not in a position to make any mistakes. Furthermore, the herbal materials kept indicating *the body can heal itself.* This created a bit of confusion, as I believed *God was going to heal me,* but the herbal program boasted *self-healing.* I asked the Lord to clarify that He was going to heal me so when my miracle arrived my message to *everyone* would be crystal clear. For two days I persisted in praying, both for a confirmation that I was doing the right thing by taking the herbs and also for the Lord to tell me it was Him and not the herbs that would perform the miracle in me.

While praying before bed on May 13, the Lord responded to my prayers with an incredible answer. I wrote it down immediately: *The herbs will not heal you, but they will prepare your body for what I am going to do. A farmer does not plant a seed in the field until he tills it, readies it, and then takes care of the field. You do likewise with your body, and I will plant the seed of marrow and it will grow a hundredfold!* I can't explain the feeling of excitement

I got after getting this word from God. It confirmed what I was doing by taking the herbs, as well as His personal involvement in a miraculous outcome!

A farmer does not plant a seed in the field until he tills it, readies it, and then takes care of the field. You do likewise with your body, and I will plant the seed of marrow and it will grow a hundredfold!

DOCTOR NOTIFIED I STOPPED TAKING MEDS

On Monday, May 14, while in for my scheduled platelet transfusion and a meeting with one of the doctors, I mentioned I had stopped taking the Cyclosporine. He was a bit surprised, but since he was a fill-in for my primary oncologist, he was not too upset by my decision. He suggested I get back on the medication right away, but I told him I was planning to get some additional opinions from other doctors over the next two weeks, as I did not think Cyclosporine was right for me.

HERBAL DETOX PROGRAM BEGINS

On Tuesday, May 15, I began a five-day herbal detoxification program designed to cleanse the colon, liver, gallbladder, blood, and a few other parts of the body. On day one I ate only fruits and vegetables. On days two through four I fasted, consuming liquids and juices only. On day five I was able to eat fruits and vegetables again.

A SECOND OPINION

On Wednesday, May 16, I made my way to the University of Minnesota Bone Marrow Transplant Center to obtain a second opinion and to discuss the nature and stipulations of a bone marrow transplant. I was also considering changing oncologists from the one I had been seeing at United Hospital and had the good fortune of meeting with an internationally renowned transplant surgeon. After reviewing my records, he agreed with the aplastic anemia diagnosis. My wife and I informed the surgeon that we did not believe a transplant would be necessary because we were expecting God to heal me miraculously without a transplant. He showed some signs of amazement but continued on with his overview of medical procedures, likely outcomes, etc.

The surgeon was hoping I'd consider using his services and the University of Minnesota Transplant Center to have the bone marrow transplant performed. There were many considerations that would ultimately lead to my making such a decision. Since I was susceptible to germs and dying at any time, they knew how important it was to find a marrow match as soon as possible. Even with a perfect match, however, the odds of a successful transplant were quite low.

I simply asked the surgeon to inform me once they located a match, or a possible match, and I would make my decision based upon the available facts at that time.

A THIRD OPINION

On Thursday, May 17, my wife and I met with another very kind, capable surgeon. He did not have anything new to say. He agreed with the diagnosis and prognosis that I had received. He said if he had been diagnosed with aplastic anemia that he would have the surgeon I just met with at the U of M perform the marrow transplant. I made a plan to visit one more doctor—a blood specialist—at the end of May.

BODY WEIGHT

For someone whose weight never changed much for years, it was interesting to see all the ups and downs in my weight in 2001!

After returning from Cancun around the first of the year, I weighed
174 pounds. During my bout with hepatitis in March, my weight
fell to 157 pounds. While in the hospital, it increased to 169 pounds
due to Prednisone, Cyclosporine, and a lack of exercise. In the two
weeks after leaving the hospital, it plummeted to 153 pounds.

BLOOD NUMBERS

May 17	My Blood Counts	Notes	Normal Range
Red	10.4	Last Transfusion: 14 Days Ago	13.5 – 17.5
White	1,000	Cannot Transfuse	3,500 – 10,800
Platelets	23,000	2 Transfusions Per Week	130,000 – 430,000
Neutrophils	0.1	Most Abundant White Cell	1.9 – 8.0

May 17: The results of my regularly scheduled blood tests are
listed above. All counts remained extremely low but no transfusions
were ordered that day. The white cell and neutrophil counts
represent the immune system and were at dangerously low levels.

PRAYER REQUESTS

As I continued to stand firmly on God's Word for my complete
healing, without a bone marrow transplant, these were my specific
prayer requests at this time:

For protection for my family and me from the enemy, as he
continues to try to sow seeds of doubt at every juncture, *for we are
not ignorant of his schemes* (2 Corinthians 2:11).

For me to cross over the goal line and score the touchdown of healing, which the Lord will perform for His glory and in His perfect timing!

For the Lord to help me in writing email updates so they touch the hearts of many: *The Spirit and bride say, 'Come'; And let the one who hears say, 'Come'; And let the one who is thirsty come; let the one who wishes take the water of life without cost* (Revelation 22:17).

CLOSING VERSES
Humble yourselves under the mighty hand of God, that He may exalt you at the proper time.

(1 Peter 5:6)

Today if you hear His voice, do not harden your hearts.

(Hebrews 4:7)

But as many as received Him, to them He gave the right to become children of God.

(John 1:12)

How will we escape if we neglect so great a salvation?

(Hebrews 2:3)

MAY 28, 2001

I had begun to feel a little better as I awaited a miraculous turnaround in my health condition. The medical world maintained that there was nothing they can do until they located a bone marrow donor. I continued to receive regular blood transfusions every three to four days.

DETOX COMPLETE
The five-day (herbal) detoxification program went well. The only complication I encountered during detox was burning the inside

of my mouth as the doses of garlic increased. I did not realize the potency of garlic—a primary ingredient in this particular cleanse—especially after juicing it in a blender. I did not rinse my mouth after drinking it, and my lips, tongue, and mouth were burned, making it very painful for several days after the program ended. Any cut or burn was a reason for alarm, as infection could easily set in, something to be avoided at all cost. Additionally, the time it would take to heal from a cut or burn is much longer when a person has a low or lacking immune system. But praise God, I was feeling better now and did not experience any infection.

There are a number of detox programs. This particular one was focused on cleansing the colon, liver, gall bladder, blood and removing any potential parasites. Each day, the program allowed for one to two SuperFood herbal drink mixes, lots of water, and plenty of juiced fruits and vegetables. I also ate bananas, asparagus, broccoli, carrots, etc. All junk food was stripped from my diet.

WHAT REALLY NEEDS TO BE DONE TO BE HEALED?

Numerous friends and recipients of my emails provided advice on what I ought to be doing in order to be healed. I received medical advice, spiritual advice, and *words from the Lord*. I appreciated the input, but the accumulation of all the advice had a tendency to become confusing. I know that *God is not a God of confusion* (1 Corinthians 14:33). So, I simply prayed for clarity, trusting my gut and following my heart with respect to whether or not I should follow any particular advice. I primarily listened to my wife and a few trusted friends whose advice I greatly respect.

What did become clear in this process of receiving advice was this: I did not need to do anything else to earn my healing. It was a done deal. In the same way that I cannot earn my salvation by being good, neither could I earn my healing by doing anything for it. I received it by faith! What began to crystallize in my mind was this: *Rejoice in the Lord always; again I will say, rejoice* (Philippians 4:4).

James 1:9 says; *But the brother of humble circumstances is to glory in his high position.* Well then, I needed to be singing praises and rejoicing, correct? Exactly! And that is just what I chose to do.

THE LATEST ON MY EYES

It was still difficult to focus properly—both up close as well as at distances. Even more bizarre than the obscured vision with my eyes open was what I saw with my eyes closed! With my eyes closed, I saw a constant image of a roaring lion! I really cannot explain this. It appeared to be in the form or substance of scar tissue. Did the scar tissue form in such a way as to create the image of a roaring lion? I doubt that. Or was I seeing a type of spiritual reflection of a Bible verse that says; *Be of sober spirit, be on the alert. Your adversary, the devil prowls around like a roaring lion, seeking someone to devour* (1 Peter 5:8)? I am more inclined to believe the latter. I sensed that I was simply being reminded that I was under spiritual attack and to *resist him, firm in faith* (1 Peter 5:9). Therefore, I was constantly speaking against the devil with authority and rebuking him so that I was not in fear of this image when I closed my eyes. And it worked!

On May 25, I made my way back to the ophthalmologist for a scheduled follow-up eye exam. I did not say anything about the image of the roaring lion. The test results showed no new damage or retinal bleeding and very slow signs that the scar tissue was dissolving. There was still a good chance that my vision could return to normal, but the doctor now felt it would take longer than the initial four-month projection.

ENEMY ATTACKS

Satan continually attempted to beat me up and wear me down. I found that the more time I would spend studying my medical diagnosis and prognosis, the more pessimistic and worrisome I had a tendency to become. It was imperative that I stood on God's Word during these times: *the Sword of the Spirit . . . is the Word of God"*

(Ephesians 6:17). The Bible is a weapon of warfare—the weapon I continued to use!

I can't emphasize this enough: if we focus on our problems in life instead of on God's promises for victory over our problems, we not only invite the enemy into our mind to remind us of our failures and our inadequacies, but we begin listening to his lies as well. I believe it is difficult to be victorious over any sickness, financial woe, relationship struggle or any other challenge if we are focusing on the problem, feeling overwhelmed and beat up. This is exactly where Satan wants us: depressed, filled with anxiety, full of doubt, and with no sense of hope. If you *want* to be set free, *allow* the Son to set you free! Abide in His Word, and you will know the truth; the truth will set you free (see John 8:31-36)!

RETURN TO THE HOSPITAL?

The oncologists and surgeons at the University of Minnesota, along with my current oncologist, recommended that I resume taking Cyclosporine to try to suppress the immune system and then undergo another round of ATG transfusions to see if there is any chance of reviving any (potential) marrow stem cells. This would mean a trip back to the hospital for a minimum of five days. The chance of success from a second ATG treatment is reduced by 50 percent. Since the first treatment produced no results, the odds of a second treatment producing any results were not good. Not only does a second attempt have less chance of success, but it also poses a higher risk of side effects. I experienced several side effects from the first treatment while in the hospital, including night-sweats, hives, heartburn, and some minor rashes. At this time, I did not feel inclined to check back into the hospital. And since no marrow donor had been found, the only option available was continued blood transfusions twice per week.

LIKE A BAD DREAM

In many ways my life could be thought of as a bad dream. Some mornings when I awoke, especially while I was in the hospital, my mind had a tendency to race through all the things the doctors told me, specifically the unfortunate outcome I would likely experience, namely death. But each day, even on an hourly basis, when negative or fearful thoughts arose, I had a choice to make. First, I chose to apply a verse from Philippians 3:13 into my life: *forgetting what lies behind and reaching forward to what lies ahead.* In addition, I chose to take *every thought captive to the obedience of Christ* (2 Corinthians 10:5). In my case, any thought that was inconsistent with a miraculous healing was taken captive and thrown out of my mind, and I continued to *walk by faith, not by sight* (2 Corinthians 5:7).

A NEW DOCTOR?

On Tuesday, May 29, I planned to meet with yet another doctor to see what he had to say about my situation. He had quite an interesting background. Although he was a chiropractor, he was also certified in herbal and homeopathic medicines, acupuncture, immune disorders, blood disorders, and several other specialties. If I understood correctly, he was only one of two such doctors in the Twin Cities with his type of training. He intended to dig into my personal background (mostly from a health perspective) to determine what may have caused my marrow and blood levels to be affected. In advance of my appointment, I had to complete a forty-five page questionnaire! This was quite a contrast from a typical new patient information form used by medical doctors.

I'M NOT GOING TO BE SICK!

My determination to be healthy and my faith that God would miraculously heal me reminded me of an experience I had many years ago. In March of 1976, when I was 19 years old and stationed in Kansas City, Missouri, in the U.S. Marine Corps, I contracted a sickness that really wore me down. My throat was incredibly sore and became infected. My tonsils, which had turned milky white in color, had swollen to the point of nearly closing off the back of my throat. I drove to the local (military) medical clinic at Richards-Gebaur Air Force Base to have it checked out. The doctor ran a few tests including a blood test. He came back and told me my white count was sky high because I had infectious mononucleosis. I asked him what we needed to do to get rid of it because tennis season was starting, and I intended to play on the Marine Corps team!

His first words were that I was not going to be playing tennis that year. I, on the other hand, intended to return to him at the next appointment in two weeks fully healed. My first stop after leaving the clinic was the public library. I remember my attitude of determination: I did not want to be sick; I wanted to play tennis. Nothing else mattered; my focus was intense. I read up on mono in the library. I wanted to learn whatever I could to fight it. After the library I went directly to the supermarket and loaded up on protein, and I called my chiropractor to set up an appointment for me to get an adjustment because I wanted my spine and the spinal fluid to flow perfectly.

On two separate occasions, while sitting up in my bed, I engaged in a mental exercise, visualizing my antibodies killing the mono cells. I returned to the doctor thirteen days after my diagnosis, and after a blood test was taken, the doctor was shocked as my blood levels were normal. Tennis season started two weeks later. For what it is worth, I went on to win the Marine Corps tournament that year for the Mid-States Region and was flown to California for a wonderful week of competitive tennis with the top Marine players in the nation. Even though I got my butt kicked, I certainly was not sick!

Now, I felt this same way. I was not going to be sick! Since I did not specifically know what my foe was this time around, it became more difficult to attack it. The big advantage I had, however, was that the Lord knew the specifics of my foe, and He fought this battle along with me. I only needed to trust Him to continue to do so.

BLOOD NUMBERS

May 24	My Blood Counts	Notes	Normal Range
Red	7.5	Last Transfusion: 21 Days Ago	13.5 – 17.5
White	800	Cannot Transfuse	3,500 – 10,800
Platelets	28,000	2 Transfusions Per Week	130,000 – 430,000
Neutrophils	0.2	Most Abundant White Cell	1.9 – 8.0

May 24: The counts from my regularly scheduled blood tests are listed above. As a result, a double-bag of red blood cells and a single bag of platelets were transfused that day.

CLOSING VERSES
For all have sinned and fall short of the glory of God.

(Romans 3:23)

For the wages of sin is death, but the free gift of God is eternal life in Christ Jesus our Lord.

(Romans 6:23)

For God so loved the world, that He gave His only begotten Son, that whoever believes in Him shall not perish, but have eternal life.

(John 3:16)

How will we escape if we neglect so great a salvation?

(Hebrews 2:3)

JUNE 3, 2001

NATURAL HOMEOPATHIC DOCTOR PASSED UP

On May 29, I went to see a *natural health* chiropractor. After our lengthy appointment and much afterthought I opted not to utilize his services. I felt like I was going to become an experiment. I know that testing is part of the fact-finding process, but after praying for discernment I sensed his experience level was not what I was looking for. I was scheduled to meet with another natural health professional on June 5. At this point, I became absolutely convinced that the natural way was right for me; I felt God leading me in that direction.

AUTOIMMUNE REVELATION!

An incredible revelation came to me with regard to suffering from an autoimmune disease. The Bible tells us the body of Christ is supposed to function and be joined together as one. As Christians, we are called to work together in unity and to build up one another in love. Ephesians 4:11-16 says; *And He gave some as apostles, and some as prophets, and some as evangelists, and some as pastors and teachers, for the equipping of the saints for the work of service, to the building up of the body of Christ; until we all attain to the unity of the faith, and of the knowledge of the Son of God, to a mature man, to the measure of the stature which belongs to the fullness of Christ. As a result, we are no longer to be children, tossed here and there by waves and carried about by every wind of doctrine, by the trickery of men, by craftiness in deceitful scheming; but speaking the truth in love, we are to grow up in all aspects into Him, who is the Head, even Christ, from whom the whole body, being fitted and held together by what every joint supplies, according to the proper working of each individual part, causes the growth of the body for the building up of itself in love.*

The body of Christ is supposed to function in harmony. Note how the analogy of the human body is used as a guide for

Christians to live and work together. Then, focus closely on the analogy itself. God's Word clearly states that the human body was designed to function in harmony with other parts of the body. If the body fails to function properly and attacks another part of the body (autoimmune), it is operating inconsistently with God's design. As Christians we have authority over the malfunctioning part of the body by commanding it to align itself in accordance with the way God created it: *For even as the body is one and yet has many members, and all the members of the body, though they are many, are one body, so also is Christ . . . for the body is not one member, but many. If the foot should say, 'Because I am not a hand, I am not a part of the body,' it is not for this reason any the less a part of the body. And if the ear should say, 'Because I am not an eye, I am not a part of the body,' it is not for this reason any the less a part of the body. If the whole body were an eye, where would the hearing be? If the whole body were hearing, where would the sense of smell be? But now God has placed members, each one of them, in the body, just as He desired . . . and now there are many members, but one body. And the eye cannot say to the hand, 'I have no need of you,' or again, the head to the feet, 'I have no need of you'* (1 Corinthians 12:12-21). So, as a result, I declared that my immune system could not say to my bone marrow, "I have no need of you."

My immune system cannot say to my bone marrow, "I have no need of you."
— JEFF SCISLOW

With these passages and the authority I have over my body, by the Word of God and its ultimate authority, I was able to address the parts of my body and command them to act in accordance with this passage from God's Word! In prayer, I commanded my immune system to never again attack the bone marrow once God restores it but rather build up and support it according to God's masterful design. More specifically, in my prayer I spoke to my immune system telling it that I was sorry for putting bad things into my body over the years, which caused it to work overtime: my poor diet, my lack of diet, and even the prescription drugs that I recently took that were designed to suppress and kill it! I then commanded my immune system to work in accordance with the way God created it, and to build up, strengthen and edify *all* parts of my body!

Wow! What a revelation God showed me! This was God's Word in action and power, and these passages spoke so clearly to my situation! I believe they will speak to anyone battling MS, rheumatoid arthritis, fibromyalgia, lupus, aplastic anemia, or any number of autoimmune diseases. And I challenge anyone with such a disorder to take authority over the attacking immune system, reminding it that it is operating against God's design and that it can no longer say to another part of your body, "I have no need of you!" Exercise your rightful authority in Christ! Know this; *For the Word of God is living and active and sharper than any two edged sword, and piercing as far as the division of soul and spirit, of joints and marrow* . . . (Hebrews 4:12). God sends out His Word and it always accomplishes what He wants; it prospers everywhere it is sent (see Isaiah 55:11).

REALTORS RESPOND!

I received a huge outpouring of love and support not only from my fellow agents at RE/MAX around the world but also from my friends in Star Power, Keller Williams, Coldwell Banker, and many other superb real estate organizations. In addition to the individual prayers of many, some added my name to their church prayer lists and others committed to praying in their small groups. I even learned I was placed on several large prayer chains of over 1,000 individuals each. That's simply awesome! As the word got out, the support continued to increase!

BLOOD NUMBERS

May 29	My Blood Counts	Notes	Normal Range
Red	9.7	Last Transfusion: 5 Days Ago	13.5 – 17.5
White	1,300	Count 5 Days Ago: 800	3,500 – 10,800
Platelets	25,000	Last Transfusion: 5 Days Ago	130,000 – 430,000
Neutrophils	0.4	Highest in 2 Months!	1.9 – 8.0

May 29: The counts from my regularly scheduled blood tests are listed above. As a result, I received a platelet transfusion. My white and neutrophil counts inched up slightly but remained at dangerous levels. There was no improvement in my vision as retinal hemorrhaging was still evident in the form of scar tissue that caused floaters and blind spots.

CLOSING VERSES

Therefore if you have been raised up with Christ, keep seeking the things above where Christ is... set your mind on the things above, not on the things that are on earth... therefore consider the members of your earthly body as dead to immorality, impurity, passion, evil desire and greed... for it is on account of these things that the wrath of God will come... put them all aside: anger, wrath, malice, slander and abusive speech from your mouth. Do not lie to one another, since you have laid aside the old self with its evil practices, and put on the new self... put on a heart of compassion, kindness, humility, gentleness and patience; bearing with one another, and forgiving each other...

just as the Lord forgave you… And beyond all these things, put on love, which is the perfect bond of unity.

(Colossians 3:1-14)

Behold, I stand at the door and knock; if anyone hears My voice and opens the door, I will come in to him, and will dine with him, and he with Me.

(Revelation 3:20)

How will we escape if we neglect so great a salvation?

(Hebrews 2:3)

JUNE 10, 2001

Day by day and hour by hour, I stayed the course. I constantly claimed: *I **will** cross over the goal line and I **will** score that touchdown!* Needless to say, the topic of healing was front and center in my life and as a result, I discovered some interesting truths these past few months.

PRINCIPLES OF HEALING

My main objective was to search the Scriptures to uncover a key principle, or principles, that would pave the way for a complete healing in my body. I explored and applied several principles of healing and continued to search for answers and revelations as I pressed on toward *perfect health in the presence of all.*

This I believe for sure: God is able to bring about a miracle any way He wishes, and it will be in accordance with His Word. As a result, my effort and strength remained focused on the variety of Biblical principles found there, particularly the ones that pertain to miraculous healing. Keep in mind these are *Christian* principles. I did not seek any other principles, although the world is filled with so many healing principles that it can make one's head spin.

PRINCIPLE ONE: FAITH ALONE

The Bible says in Hebrews 11:6; *And without faith it is impossible to please Him, for he that comes to God must believe that He is and that He is a rewarder of those who seek Him.* God promises to reward those who diligently seek Him in faith. I believe that the promise in this verse alone is enough to bring forth and manifest any healing. Hebrews 11:1 states; *Now faith is the assurance of things hoped for, the conviction of things not seen.* This means simply believing, without wavering, in that which we expect to happen, even though it has not yet occurred or physically materialized.

In Mark chapter 9, beginning at verse 17, we learn of a father who brought his demon-possessed son before Jesus to be healed. A very important aspect of exercising one's faith takes place here. The boy's father states he believes but needs help with his unbelief. In response Jesus says that all things are possible to those who believe. Note, that the boy's father asks Jesus to help his *unbelief.* I see this as an illustration of where God performs miracles and heals even if our faith is not perfect! Why? Because *Jesus is the author and perfecter of our faith* (Hebrews 12:2). Jesus perfects our faith before God the Father on our behalf! The boy's father had a pure heart, spoke truthfully, sought Jesus' help, and Jesus honored his request.

Believing is crucial, but even in our weakness (as it relates to faith) God is able and willing to move miraculously. This boy was healed because his father acted on faith alone, and even though the father admitted his faith might be short of God's expectations, God honored the sincerity of his heart, had compassion on him, and healed his son.

PRINCIPLE TWO:
CONDITIONAL UPON AN ACTION

The issue of self-examination is not necessarily a topic we look forward to, but it is one that I believe is very important to receiving breakthroughs in our lives. The Apostle Paul spoke to the Corinthians about this—how failure to examine themselves was resulting in many of them being sick and even dying: *many among you are weak and sick, and a number sleep. But if we judged ourselves rightly, we would not be judged* (1 Corinthians 11:28-31).

The topic of self-examination, and the subsequent repentance of any sin as a condition to receive healing, is explored in detail in a book I read by Pastor Henry Wright, *A More Excellent Way—A Teaching on the Spiritual Roots of Disease*. The book makes it clear that conditions may exist in our lives that can prevent healing and miracles from manifesting, and once certain conditions are met, spiritual doors are unlocked to receive the miraculous.

As I read through the introduction, I was challenged to search my heart and ask God if there was anything in my life that needed repentance, anything that might have possibly brought this affliction upon me, or *anything* that was standing in the way of my being healed. I was determined to examine and judge myself rightly!

PRINCIPLE THREE:
CALLING IT INTO EXISTENCE

I also read a wonderful book by Charles Capps called *God's Creative Power for Healing*. His book taught me several powerful concepts: healing promises from God's Word, which are spiritual in nature, will heal the physical body as it is applied on a regular basis; voicing God's Word in faith establishes what God has promised even if physical healing has not yet manifested; when you confess that you are healed by Jesus' stripes you are simply calling for healing that God has already provided; and your words have more effect on your body than anyone else's. These concepts are in line with Proverbs 18:21, which says, *Life and death are in the power of the tongue!*

After reading Capps' book, I made the decision to write out over thirty affirmations and demands according to the Word of God and His covenant/promise for healing. I used large sticky notes and put them around the house so that I could see them often during the day. I *spoke them out loud* regularly and with authority.

MY STICKY NOTE AFFIRMATIONS

Jesus
came to
give LIFE
and give it
Abundantly!
Thank-you
Lord.!!

I thank you
Lord
for full &
complete
Healing!
According to Thy
Word...
I'm healed!

And this is
the VICTORY
that overcomes
the world —
My Faith!

Thank you
Father for
the Fresh,
Powerful &
healthy
Bone Marrow!

I know the plans I have for you saith the Lord — Plans for Hope and for a Future!

"Let there be Marrow!" And it was granted unto him according to his Faith!

Jesus has Set me Free from the Law of Sin and Death!

My body is the temple of the Holy Spirit, where NO darkness or disease can dwell!

My
Immune System
shall support
all other
organs, cells
and every fiber
in my body
(I Corin 12)

NO
Weapon
formed against
Me
shall prosper!

(Isa 54:17)

The Lord
has delivered
me from every
Kind of
sickness & disease!

I'm healed!

The hand cannot
say to the foot
"I don't need you"

The eye cannot
say to the ear
"I don't need you"

nor can...

The immune system
say to the bone marrow
"I don't need you"

(I Corin 12)

And the man said, "Lord, if thou will, Ye can make me whole." And Jesus said, "I WILL"

Greater is He who is in Me than he who is in the world (I John 4:4)

By Jesus' STRIPES I'm Healed (I Peter 2:24)

I Bind All Sickness and Disease that shall come Against me in the Name of Jesus, and cast it into the Pit!

NUTRITION & NATURAL SUBSTANCES

I have read a lot about how the body can heal itself. God created our bodies to function victoriously when under attack from a variety of viruses, bacteria, etc. I believe this even more so since becoming sick. I read *Live Right 4 Your Type* by Dr. Peter D'Adamo, a book that teaches how our bodies chemically react to what we eat and drink based upon our individual blood type. According to D'Adamo's book, I was eating a variety of foods that are not best suited for my blood type, so I made yet another adjustment. Clearly, I was very teachable at this stage. From food to herbs and from lifestyle to spiritual matters, I was open and seeking the Lord for His guidance.

GENERATIONAL CURSES & DELIVERANCE

The Bible says God will visit the iniquities of the fathers on the children and on the grandchildren to the third and fourth generations (Exodus 20:5; 34:7; Numbers 14:18; Deuteronomy 5:9). My wife and I met with Marjorie Cole, a lecturer, counseling minister, and author of *Taking the Devil to Court* to discuss generational curses. Marjorie has exceptional insight into this often-overlooked area of Scripture. We learned a lot in the two hours we spent together, even though we only touched on the surface of this deep subject. As an example of her knowledge and insight, she ascertained with certainty that I had royalty in my blood, simply due to the doctor's diagnosis. I had actually forgotten that I was related to Queen Elizabeth! She pointed out that many blood disorders have been passed down through the generations within royal families. I found this most interesting, as I was familiar with Bible passages which indicate certain diseases are the results of generational curses.

My grandmother on my dad's side died of a blood disorder. I never met her; she died the year I was born at roughly the same age I was when I was diagnosed!

GETTING OUT AND ABOUT

I made a bold decision to start getting out of the house and to trust God to protect me from germs. I watched my boys' soccer games and went shopping for the first time since I was discharged from the hospital. I even went on several listing appointments in other people's homes! In the natural mind it was scary, if not outright crazy, but I concluded that I must live as though I will live, not as though I will die. I prayed for protection and asked God to keep me at home if I was acting irresponsibly. Since I had peace about this, I ventured out, without a mask of course!

I even went on listing appointments in other people's homes . . . I did not want to be foolish; dying as a result of stupidity would have been a terrible way to go!

When I ventured out of the house, it was like walking out on a branch of a tree, going a little further, and then a little further and trusting God to keep the branch from breaking. I did not want to be foolish; dying as a result of stupidity would have been a terrible way to go. I kept my hands clean with hand sanitizer and always prayed that God would keep me from accidentally rubbing my eyes or touching my nose or mouth with my hands.

BLOOD NUMBERS NOT HOLDING

I still needed regular blood transfusions. On June 4, I decided to conduct my own little test and told my oncologist to skip the scheduled platelet transfusion that day so I could see if my body would produce platelets if in dire need. Surprised at my request, he warned against this since my platelet count had already fallen to a level that clearly warranted a transfusion. I told him it was only for three days, and since he could not force me to get the platelet transfusion, he reluctantly agreed to my experiment.

I knew it was in my best interest to get as few transfusions as possible because my body could be building a resistance to transfused blood. If this were the case, my body could reject additional transfusions at any point and leave me with little time to live. Since fewer transfusions are better, and since I wanted to see if my body would produce more platelets if they were seriously needed, I proceeded to skip this one scheduled transfusion and recheck my platelet count in three days.

On June 7, my platelet count was nearly depleted! It was not only disappointing that the platelets had not held at all, but it was also very dangerous and could have resulted in internal bleeding. An immediate platelet transfusion was ordered. Because the platelet level had fallen so low, the doctors ordered some additional blood tests that day to ensure I had not brought on any new complications.

DOCTOR UPDATE

I spent a great deal of time seeking out doctors and medical advice. I wanted to work with professionals with whom I was comfortable, who took an interest in me, and who I felt knew what they were doing. The results of my findings, based on the various professional groups, follow:

- Western: I saw four oncology/specialists from the Western medical profession and all completely agreed with my diagnosis and prognosis. None of these doctors offered any new ideas or suggestions for a different treatment. All recommended that I submit to another round of ATG transfusions and undergo a bone marrow transplant, providing a suitable donor was located.

- Naturopathic: Naturopathy is "a system of treatment of diseases that avoids drugs and surgery and emphasizes the use of natural agents (such as air, water, and herbs) and physical means (such as tissue manipulation and electrotherapy)" (*The Merriam-Webster Dictionary*). I went to two naturopaths after being discharged from the hospital. The first was neutral, neither optimistic nor pessimistic. He seemed less educated than I had hoped, and I feared I might become an experiment in an area in which he was perhaps unfamiliar. The second seemed laid back, tired, and somewhat disinterested although he had extensive knowledge. Both my wife and I were concerned about his office, which was a melting pot of religious books and figurines from Hinduism to Taoism; from New Age to Buddhism and more. Both naturopaths seemed indifferent to my diagnosed illness. I felt like a number, a non-issue.

- Herbal: I visited a Chinese herbal and acupuncture specialist who was familiar with aplastic anemia. She asked some of the same questions as the Western medical doctors to try to determine how I might have contracted it. She also carefully examined my blood reports and tests and gave me some herbs to boost my blood and energy levels, but, like the others, she did not seem optimistic about my recovery. She repeatedly cautioned me to take care of myself and to avoid exposure to anyone that was ill. She was more concerned than all of the other professionals I saw, showing great empathy but lacking optimism.

- Spiritual: Marjorie Cole had a different perspective than any of the others. Both my wife and I were interested in hearing more about what she had to say. She felt that a crack in my spiritual armor may have occurred resulting in the release of a generational curse. She felt I might have been in need of deliverance from a spirit that had attacked and oppressed me physically. Knowledgeable in the area of spiritual warfare and deliverance, Marjorie also showed concern for me and was the only person who expressed optimism for healing through prayer and deliverance.

PROPHETIC MESSAGES

I had several pastors and prophetic ministers deliver messages that were anywhere from interesting to bizarre. In each case, it was important for me to discern the message. One such bizarre message came in the form of a letter addressed to me, written by a so-called prophetess. In the long letter, the woman told me that God would only heal me if I helped her and her family financially—failing to do so would result in my death. After I discussed it with my wife and close friends, I prayed about it and ended up throwing the letter out. I chose not to believe these words since they brought only fear, and her letter was inconsistent with God's Word. The message from Pastor Steve Munsey, however, *There is someone here tonight who the doctors have told does not have long to live; God is going to remove that sickness; and add fifteen years to your life,* proved to be one of my most interesting messages. Unlike the one from the *prophetess*, this message was consistent with God's Word and produced joy in me and not fear.

QUIET TIME WITH GOD

I needed to be quiet before God on a regular basis and just listen. While spending time with Him, I was given peace that I would be healed. That is all I really needed, isn't it? So I simply stepped out of the busyness of the day and learned to be quiet and listen. He loves it when His kids do that!

BLOOD NUMBERS

June 7	My Blood Counts	Notes	Normal Range
Red	8.4	Last Transfusion: 14 Days Ago	13.5 – 17.5
White	1,400	Count 3 Days Ago: 1,000	3,500 – 10,800
Platelets	3,000	Last Transfusion: 9 Days Ago	130,000 – 430,000
Neutrophils	0.4	Most Abundant White Cell	1.9 – 8.0

June 7: The counts from my regularly scheduled blood tests are listed above. The platelets had fallen to a dangerously low level as a result of my failed experiment and an immediate transfusion was ordered. A double-bag of red blood cells was ordered and transfused the following day. As of this date, 153 tubes of blood had been drawn since the onset of the illness. Scar tissue from the retinal hemorrhaging was still evident, causing blind spots in my vision. My daily weight ranged between 154 and 156 pounds.

CLOSING VERSES
For this is the love of God, that we keep His commandments and His commandments are not burdensome.

(1 John 5:3)

Let us not love with word or with tongue, but in deed and truth. We will know by this that we are of the truth, and will assure our heart before Him, in whatever our heart condemns us; for God is greater than our heart and knows all things. If our heart does not condemn us, we have confidence before God; and whatever we ask we receive from Him, because we keep His commandments and do the things which are pleasing in His sight.

(1 John 3:18-22)

How will we escape if we neglect so great a salvation?

(Hebrews 2:3)

JULY 6, 2001

In early June I began venturing outdoors to watch the soccer games of my seven and nine-year-old boys. As I did, I became more comfortable with normal living, even in the absence of an immune system! Soon, I was going to church again, eating at restaurants occasionally, and, of course, I had been going on real estate appointments. The doctors thought I was crazy getting out in public this way, but I chose to live like a man who was going to live and not like one who planned to die! Praise God for His protection, and the peace and assurance He provided me. I will never forget His promise: *After you have suffered for a little while, the God of all grace, who called you to His eternal glory in Christ, shall Himself, restore, strengthen, perfect, establish and confirm you* (1 Peter 5:10).

ANALOGY: A TORNADO OR A FLOOD?

I have long pondered the question of whether the diagnosis of aplastic anemia was the result of something resembling a "tornado" or a "flood" hitting my body. Let me explain. A tornado's characteristics are that it arrives unexpectedly and swiftly, doing major damage. Then just as quickly as it appeared it is gone—nowhere to be found. In contrast, a flood's characteristics are that it arrives slowly and its presence continues to do damage by putting pressure on the affected area. So which scenario best describes this disease?

I shared this analogy with my doctors, asking whether the nature of the disease resembled the tornado or the flood, and I never got a response. The doctors did not know, and the naturopaths did not know—none of the professionals I spoke to knew. But it was significant to me because, the way I see it, treating a disease that swiftly hit the body and is now *gone* (tornado) should be quite different than treating the same disease that is *still present* (flood). How can any treatment be prescribed if the doctors cannot answer this question?

If my marrow was hit as if by a flood, and if this so-called flood was still present and still putting pressure on my bone marrow, then natural immune system boosters—like Echinacea, MGN-3, and Goldenseal—would only add to the pressure on any marrow that might exist now or in the future by enhancing *natural killer cells* to kill it. Instead of enhancing the immune system, taking such boosters would ensure the marrow remained under attack by these natural killer cells, and would prevent any improvement to the immune system. On the other hand, if my marrow was hit hard and damaged as if by a tornado, resulting in a greatly reduced white cell count, then those same immune system boosters could benefit me by strengthening and protecting me from germs, infections, and their associated life-threatening complications.

MGN-3 is not well known by many, including the medical doctors who cared for me. It is a relatively new immune system enhancer that boosts the effectiveness of the natural killer cells by 300 percent (not in numbers but in activity levels). It also modulates and regulates the immune system and has proven to be a wonderful supplement for fighting cancers, since many cancers develop as the result of a weakened immune system. This product could have potentially boosted the effectiveness of the few white natural killer cells being produced in my lymph nodes, thymus and spleen.

In my investigation into MGN-3, I repeatedly attempted to reach the research scientist who developed the product. I left several detailed messages for him but never received a call back. I hoped to ask him what he knew about aplastic anemia and whether he believed MGN-3 would be beneficial or detrimental for someone who has been diagnosed with the disease. I did successfully reach two different product managers at Lane Labs, the company that manufactures MGN-3. I presented my flood and tornado scenarios to them, but neither had an idea as to whether their product might be helpful for a person having been diagnosed with aplastic anemia. They advised that I do more homework before trying the supplement. I agreed with them, as I felt the risk of taking MGN-3 outweighed the potential benefit at this point.

HEAVY METAL (NOT ROCK 'N' ROLL)

In late June, I met for a second time with one of the naturopaths I met earlier in the month. We discussed heavy metal toxicity and the chance that aplastic anemia could be the result of exposure to some type of heavy metal or other toxin. We decided to find out. We sent hair samples from the back of my neck to a laboratory in Chicago for analysis. A few days later, the naturopath called telling me the levels of aluminum and tin in my system were very high. The aluminum build-up most likely occurred from standard antiperspirant usage over the years. We have no idea why the tin levels were so high. In either case, there was no immediate cause for alarm based on this preliminary report. A comprehensive report with any recommendations would arrive within a week or so.

While studying toxicity, I learned that benzene is the only substance listed on the Centers for Disease Control's most dangerous substance list that attacks bone marrow. I'm not aware of

any possible exposure to benzene, but I found it interesting that it
attacks bone marrow in particular.

BACK PAIN HEALED

Also at the end of June, a friend felt directed by the Lord to tell
me to take my family out of town for a day or two, just to get away. I
considered this a great idea, and my family and I made plans to drive
about an hour south to Lake City for the day. We planned to leave
around 10:00 a.m. An hour before departure time, I ran to Rainbow
Foods to pick up not two, not four, but ten forty-pound bags of salt
for the water softener. Although I had been feeling good, I had not
exercised in quite some time. I loaded all ten bags into the shopping
cart, wheeled them out to my truck and proceeded home. From
the truck, I carried the bags one at a time down to the basement
of my home and into the utility room. Feeling good, and with only
two bags to go, I jerked them out of the back of the truck in one
motion, one in each hand. As I caught the weight of those last two
bags, the middle of my back nearly gave out. I continued into the
house, carrying them down the steps into the basement. Halfway
across the basement floor, I suddenly froze and dropped the bags
as a sharp pain exploded in my back. I could not take another step.

Forgetting about the salt bags lying on the floor, I eventually
managed to get up the steps to the main floor where I carefully sat
down in a chair. The pain was awful. I was brought an ice pack and
rested on the couch. I could barely move. Before long, my kids were
asking me to go. Unable to acknowledge their request, I just laid
there immobile and in pain. My wife told the kids that Dad had hurt
his back and that we would just stay home today and go another
time. The kids were quite disappointed.

I prayed right there on the couch saying, *Lord, I am sorry. I
really messed up. I have felt pretty good lately and I was not thinking. I
was not in shape to haul all that salt and then manhandle two bags at
a time. It was stupid! I am sorry. I know that You wanted me to take*

this trip with the family today—to have fun and get away. I need Your help now. In Jesus' name I ask that you loosen the muscles in my back so that I can get up and go with the family. I trust You and thank You! Praise Thy name! Amen! I had thrown my back out several times in the past; I knew how painful it was, and I knew it could take several days to several weeks to get back to normal. I tell you this most truly: ten minutes after praying, I slowly got up from the couch. I carefully walked around, praising God. I walked outside. I gently took steps so that I did not pull any more back muscles. The looser I felt, the more I praised God! I was ready to try to get up into the truck; I pulled myself up, I got out of the truck, I got in it again, and I got out again. My back was tender, but the contracted muscles had loosened! We loaded the kids in the truck and hit the road!

My family had a blast spending the day together. It was not only a treat to get away with everyone but also to be reminded that God was there with us and that He made it all possible. It was terrific having the healing prayer for my back answered so quickly and I truly wanted the same quick results with regard to the disease that was threatening my life. God had acted in His perfect timing to heal my back on this day and I trusted the same perfect timing would take place in my being healed from aplastic anemia. In a way, waiting for that healing was difficult, yet in another way it was not. I had such an assurance in God's promises for me that I was not all that concerned as to how long it might take for a full and complete healing to arrive. As long as I stayed the course and demonstrated faith and patience along the way I knew I would receive the healing I sought.

HEALING ROOMS

While in the hospital, I read a book about John G. Lake, an incredible man who was born in Canada in 1870. Among other significant accomplishments, he founded the Healing Rooms of Spokane in Washington. The Healing Rooms were a special place where people could go to receive prayer. The anointed prayer warriors, or *technicians*, saw and prayed for 200 people per day on average! Spokane hospitals began closing down because so many people were being healed. God was moving powerfully through Lake's ministry. As a result, Spokane was officially named the healthiest city in the USA.

After Lake passed away, the healing rooms soon went by the wayside, until more recently when they reopened in Spokane. Since the reopening, other ministries have gone to Spokane and have had their prayer ministers trained under the guidelines and principles that John G. Lake developed in the mid-twentieth century. One such ministry is Healing Center International, located in the Twin Cities.

My wife and I have visited this ministry three times. Each time, we were blessed to have intelligent, well-trained Christian counselors listen to us, ask lots of questions, and then pray for exactly what we needed. There was a genuine desire to get to the root of problems and to come against them in Jesus' name, expecting the Lord to move and heal (whether physical, emotional, spiritual, or financial).

BLOOD NUMBERS—A CLOSE LOOK

On July 5, my blood numbers reached new heights in three major categories—white count, platelets, and neutrophils! In addition to seeing these new highs, I noticed something extremely interesting in my blood test results that date back to when I began taking herbs and received the word from the Lord about tilling, readying, and taking care of the field.

Since my journey began, whenever my white count hit a new high, it always fell back again, usually on the next test. Now, for the first time my white count stayed steady. It did not fall back after hitting a new high. In fact, on July 2, my white count hit 1,700 and remained at 1,700 for my July 5 test. These were the highest white counts produced since I was diagnosed with aplastic anemia. My average white count was just 500 during the month of April. In May, the average increased to 925. In June, it inched up to 1,250. In July, the average was 1,700! The normal white count range is between 3,500 and 10,800. So, I was halfway to reaching the normal range.

My platelet count was higher also, reaching 51,000! I either received some incredible platelets, or my counts were simply holding very well—perhaps it was a combination.

Neutrophils are the most abundant type of white blood cells in humans and form an integral part of the immune system. My average neutrophil count was 0.0 during the month of April. In May, the average increased slightly to 0.15. In June, the average was 0.385. On July 5, the count hit 0.60—a new high! The normal neutrophil count range is 1.9 to 8.0. This new count put me a third of the way to a normal level.

While at my oncologist's clinic waiting for a blood transfusion, I noticed a particular set of blood numbers from the collection of my CBC (Complete Blood Count) tests that showed a significant change. The blood numbers I described above are *quantity* numbers, or blood counts. Mine, of course, were well below normal. The significant change I noticed was not in the blood counts however, but in the balance of the overall immune system. The percentages of all white cells (the immune system) were improving!

The few white blood cells that I had in my body were being produced in the lymph nodes, thymus and spleen. These organs only produce about 5 percent of what is needed for a healthy immune system, while bone marrow (if present) produces 95 percent. Even though a very small quantity of white cells existed, the percentage *quality* of these different white cells within my overall immune system was improving.

The immune system is made up of several different types of white cells. The three most predominant types are neutrophils, lymphocytes, and monocytes. These three white cell types comprise nearly the entire white cell allocation (immune system). In a healthy immune system, the neutrophil white cells comprise approximately 65 percent of all white cells, the lymphocyte white cells comprise approximately 25 percent of all white cells, and the monocyte white cells comprise up to 10 percent of all white cells.

At the time I was admitted into the hospital, my CBC test results clearly indicated that my neutrophil percentage was nowhere near the normal range. It continued to get worse and worse, that is, until I stopped the Cyclosporine, began taking herbs, and received a confirmation from the Lord on May 13. My neutrophil percentage had fallen all the way to 7.4 percent on May 10. It then turned 180 degrees and began rising, posting a percentage of 11.9 percent on May 14 and 15.0 percent on May 17! It continued to rise slowly back toward normal levels, as evidenced by each new CBC. On July 5, the percentage climbed to 35.7 percent! The normal range is 45.0 to 76.0 percent. This was amazing!

Similarly, the lymphocyte percentage was elevated and out of balance when I was admitted into the hospital. It continued to worsen until I stopped the Cyclosporine, began taking herbs, and received a confirmation from the Lord on May 13. My lymphocyte percentage soared all the way to 83.4 percent on May 10, and then turned 180 degrees and began falling, posting a percentage of 75.5 percent on May 14 and 64.3 percent on May 17! It continued to fall slowly back toward normal levels, as evidenced by each new CBC test. On July 5, the percentage was down to 50.6 percent. The normal range is 15.0 to 43.0 percent.

I felt very excited over this discovery! Something good was happening, and I believed it was due to the herbs the Lord directed me to take. Once the soil (of my body) was tilled, readied, and taken care of, the Lord promised to plant the seed of marrow, and that it would grow a hundredfold!

After my blood transfusion, I located my oncologist and enthusiastically showed him the changes I noticed from my CBC test results dating back to May. With a mundane voice he said, "That does not matter. You don't have any bone marrow."

I said, "No, it *does* matter; something is happening here!"

He responded, "I am sorry. You don't have any marrow," and continued walking down the hall.

Disappointed that my doctor was not excited, I felt a bit discouraged during my drive home from the clinic. Before long, however, I gathered my thoughts and chose to believe that the change in the quality of my white cell composition was a big deal, even if the quantity was not there yet. I knew it was coming!

The following chart indicates a substantial improvement in the *percentages* of my primary white blood cells:

White Cell Percentages	May 10	July 5	Normal Range
Neutrophils	7.4%	35.7%	45.0 – 76.0%
Lymphocytes	83.4%	50.6%	15.0 – 43.0%
Monocytes	19.6%	12.0%	0.0 – 10.0%

There are only two known medical ways to beat aplastic anemia. One is a successful ATG treatment and the other is a successful bone marrow transplant. In my case, the ATG treatment failed and no known marrow donor existed. As a result, the doctors said it was only a matter of time before I died from this disease. I have been unable to find an account of anyone recovering from aplastic anemia without success from one of these two procedures.

BLOOD NUMBERS

July 5	My Blood Counts	Notes	Normal Range
Red	10.2	Last Transfusion: 9 Days Ago	13.5 – 17.5
White	1,700	Count 3 Days Ago: 1,700	3,500 – 10,800
Platelets	51,000	Last Transfusion: 3 Days Ago	130,000 – 430,000
Neutrophils	0.6	Count 3 Days Ago: 0.5	1.9 – 8.0

July 5: The counts from my regularly scheduled blood tests are listed above. The white count, platelets, and neutrophils improved but were a considerable ways from normal. Even with this slight improvement, the oncologist assured me there was no bone marrow in my body. As of this date, 167 tubes of blood had been drawn since the onset of the illness. Scar tissue from the retinal hemorrhaging was still evident and continued to cause blind spots in my vision.

CLOSING VERSES

Heal me, O Lord, and I will be healed; save me and I will be saved, for You are my praise.

(Jeremiah 17:14)

Come to Me, all who are weary and heavy-laden, and I will give you rest. Take My yoke upon you, and learn from Me, for I am gentle and humble in heart; and you will find rest for your souls. For My yoke is easy, and My burden is light.

(Matthew 11:28-30)

How will we escape if we neglect so great a salvation?

(Hebrews 2:3)

JULY 16, 2001

On Thursday, July 12, my blood numbers inched their way to the highest levels since the onset of this disease. While these levels were still a long way from normal, I was staying positive and expecting a miraculous, 100-percent recovery in spite of the doctors telling me otherwise.

I was diligent to keep my little bottle of liquid antibacterial hand sanitizer with me; after shaking hands with someone, I would quickly cleanse. Although not a bad practice for anyone to incorporate into his or her daily life, it was an essential one for me; I didn't need to land back in the hospital or die because of a cold or flu.

With respect to the business, my wife was primarily focusing on phones and client files in the office, and I was back out on appointments. The doctor warned against my going back to work, but I sensed the proverbial branch was strong so I kept stepping out further and further with the faith that I was protected from getting sick. Although my blood numbers are inching upward, I did not have an immune system capable of fighting off an invading germ— yet! I had further to go, but I was getting there and would cross over that goal line exactly as God revealed to me. I simply could not put into words the joy, excitement, and anticipation I was experiencing as I believed the manifestation of the miracle was so close.

HEAVY METAL CHELATION SCHEDULED

We still had no idea why my levels of tin were so high. Speculating it could be resulting from our house water, we arranged to have my wife's hair analyzed as well. In our efforts to provide a healthy environment at home, we purchased a whole house water filtration system. Although we had a good municipal water system, toxins could have still been present. And since toxins can be absorbed through skin, the body's largest organ, we opted for the water filtration system. We now enjoy bottle-quality water from every faucet and shower in the house.

Chelation therapy is defined, in part, as a process that "binds metals (such as lead or iron) in the body to form a chelation so that the metal loses its toxic effect or physiological activity and is eventually passed through and out of the body" (*The Merriam-Webster Dictionary*). The naturopathic doctor and I discussed the various chelation options at my previous appointment. While the intravenous method is quicker and more complete than the oral (supplemental) method, its cost was much higher, and the chelation sessions had to be administered at the naturopathic doctor's office. I chose the oral method and ordered my first supply of chelation supplements.

The oral chelation process can take up to six months to complete. The process begins with liver and bladder cleansing. These organs need to be strong, healthy, and cleaned out so they can begin receiving the heavy metal toxins that pass through them as they are eliminated from my body.

There were no major side effects expected, since I was to begin the supplements gradually, taking the chelating supplements every other day and working up to three times per day. This was to help avoid overloading my liver or bladder with heavy metals. After three months, I would get another hair analysis to determine how well the chelation program was working.

BACK TO CHURCH
On July 15, I attended another regular church service; the third one since early April when I was admitted to the hospital. With the past two visits to church, I left just before the service ended because I was not supposed to be in large crowds due to the chance of infection. I felt more comfortable this time so I stayed after and talked with anyone who wanted to say hello and get a firsthand

update on my health progress. This was a very special time for me, and I felt blessed to be able to visit with so many of my friends.

SUNDAY'S SERMON: THE PRINCIPLE OF THE SEED

During the church service, Pastor Dave Housholder, one of the Hosanna Church pastors, discussed Genesis 26:12. This verse says, *Now Isaac sowed in that land and reaped in the same year a hundredfold. And the Lord blessed him.* I immediately felt the parallel of this verse with what the Lord spoke to my heart during my prayer on May 13. The Lord had said that if I tilled the soil (of my body) by eating right, taking care of it, and by taking the herbs, He Himself would plant the seed of marrow, and it would grow a hundredfold! That meant no drugs, no medications, and no transplants—hallelujah! With the blood counts on the rise, I believed the Lord has already planted the seed of marrow and that it was growing.

I always believed my healing would arrive, but I did not know when. I continued to see a marked increase in the blood numbers, especially those crucial white counts. Yet I did not hear anything from the oncologist about my improving test results. The nurses, however, were beginning to unofficially acknowledge them, and, as they did, I reminded them that this was the miracle I had been talking about.

TESTING THE BODY'S ENDURANCE

Although I felt excellent and looked much better, my true physical condition had been weakened as a result of not exercising regularly; being sick with hepatitis during February and March; being confined in a hospital room for twenty-eight days in April; and being instructed by my doctor to refrain from any physical activity after being released from the hospital in May.

I did simple exercises such as sit-ups and light dumbbell curls. While doing these, I would pay close attention to my need for oxygen (anemic responses). My breathing felt good, but my muscles tired quickly, either from lack of exercise, lack of oxygen to the muscles, or both.

Since the oxygen to my lungs felt adequate, I pushed myself a bit more to see how my body would react to exercise. I took my mountain bike down from the ceiling hooks in the garage, pumped up the tires, and went on an eight mile bike ride (on pavement) in 90-degree heat. Although I had not biked since the previous year, I did not feel anemic. I praised God because I knew that my hemoglobin was finally strong enough to produce the oxygen needed for such a ride!

Knowing that I had the energy to ride a bike, I wanted to test my ability to jog. I was quickly reminded that jogging is more demanding than riding a bike; I tired quickly and experienced both shortness of breath and a rapid depletion of leg muscle strength. My calves, shins, and thighs began to fall asleep from a lack of oxygen after only a one block jog. If I would have continued, I would have fallen since my legs had no more energy for additional steps. I had my work cut out for me and planned to keep exercising and believing in higher and higher blood counts in the days ahead.

BLOOD NUMBERS—A CLOSE LOOK

On July 12, my blood numbers were mixed. Both the hemoglobin and platelet cells continued to deplete slowly, and I required both red cell and platelet transfusions. However, the white count inched upward to a new high of 1,800! With the normal range being between 3,500 and 10,800, I was halfway to a normal level of white cells. Since the white cell count was increasing, I believed something must be happening in the bone marrow!

My neutrophils—the predominant white cells within the immune system—also inched upward to 0.70. With the normal range being between 1.9 and 8.0, I was more than a third of the way to a normal level. While in the hospital, my neutrophil counts were

0.0 when the doctors confirmed I had no bone marrow or stem cells.

I also continued to see healthier percentages (quality) of the three primary types of white cells—neutrophils, lymphocytes, and monocytes. They were all moving toward the normal range. The change is depicted in the following chart:

White Cell Percentages	May 10	July 5	July 12	Normal Range
Neutrophils	7.4%	35.7%	41.0%	45.0 – 76.0%
Lymphocytes	83.4%	50.6%	44.1%	15.0 – 43.0%
Monocytes	19.6%	12.0%	13.4%	0.0 – 10.0%

BLOOD NUMBERS

July 12	My Blood Counts	Notes	Normal Range
Red	10.0	Last Transfusion: 16 Days Ago	13.5 – 17.5
White	1,800	Count 7 Days Ago: 1,700	3,500 – 10,800
Platelets	20,000	Last Transfusion: 7 Days Ago	130,000 – 430,000
Neutrophils	0.7	Count 7 Days Ago: 0.6	1.9 – 8.0

July 12: The counts from my regularly scheduled blood tests are listed above. The white count and neutrophils improved ever so slightly, while the hemoglobin and platelets declined. My blood

draw count reached 169 tubes, and my daily weight was steady and ranged between 155 and 156 pounds. I had an appointment with the ophthalmologist on July 12 and was told my eyes look wonderful. The retinal scarring from the hemorrhages were dissolving and getting thinner. He expected them to be gone soon. The surface area of the scar tissue had not changed, but the depth of the scarring was decreasing. Once the scar tissue completely dissolved, light would pass perfectly through my eyes, and my vision would be completely restored. Since some of the scar tissue still remained, I had some minor blind spots but could no longer see the image of the roaring lion. He was in the process of being totally defeated!

CLOSING VERSES

Do not be deceived . . . Every good thing given and every perfect gift is from above, coming down from the Father of lights, with whom there is no variation, or shifting shadow.

(James 1:16-17)

For all flesh is like grass, and all its glory like the flower of grass. The grass withers, and the flower falls off, but the Word of the Lord endures forever...

(1 Peter 1:24-25)

How will we escape if we neglect so great a salvation?"

(Hebrews 2:3)

AUGUST 1, 2001

A WORD OF HEALING

On July 19, I received the following prophetic word from a fellow believer who I did not know at the time and who I have yet to meet. Ginger, a RE/MAX real estate agent from South Carolina who had been receiving my email updates, blessed me with the following email note on Thursday, July 19:

Sometimes I hear from God very clearly. Today, while I was playing a computer game, I heard God say this to me: *Tell Jeff he has endeared himself to Me. I have healed many of disease, including aplastic anemia, and very few have expressed such high levels of gratitude and praise to Me.* Jeff, it reminded me of when Jesus healed the ten lepers and only one returned to thank Him. Jeff, you are His beloved.

Ginger

Tell Jeff he has endeared himself to Me. I have healed many of disease, including aplastic anemia, and very few have expressed such high levels of gratitude and praise to Me.

WARNINGS, WARNINGS, WARNINGS

I often reflect back on what it was like living in the hospital and the daily visits from my oncologist, who constantly reminded me of my body's weakened and susceptible state. During my twenty-eight-day stay as a resident of United Hospital, my white blood cell count fluctuated in a dangerous range of 200 to 800 (3,500 to 10,800 is normal). Since the risk of viral, bacterial, or fungal infection was critically high, many precautions were necessary. I was required to wear a mask whenever I had a visitor. Visitors had to wash their hands before entering the room and either wear a gown or keep their distance from me. I could not shake hands or hug anyone. All flowers or fruits I received from loved ones were confiscated due to the risk of an airborne infection.

Then the warnings became even more bizarre and detailed. Instructions on the bathroom wall provided advice on which direction to wipe myself after a bowel movement to lessen the chances of bleeding. Other bathroom instructions detailed how to rinse my mouth after meals with a baking soda and salt formula they prepared for me. I was instructed to brush my teeth gently with a feather-like toothbrush to prevent my gums from bleeding.

The doctor informed me that most aplastic anemia patients die from complications (colds, flu, pneumonia, etc.) from being in what others consider a normal environment and that I best be careful. When I inquired about the possibility of going out on real estate appointments, I was advised not to do so because of differing germs and not knowing whether someone in a particular house was sick. When I asked about attending church, they recommended against it since there were too many people around. In addition, I needed to always keep a thermometer nearby to frequently check my temperature. If it rose to 101 degrees, I needed to immediately return to the hospital for possible treatment. The warnings seemed to never end and the dismal prognosis weighed heavy on me.

It was easy to get depressed by all this information. At times I thought that I might as well have just stayed in the hospital. Undoubtedly, this was a challenging time. How I responded however was totally up to me, and I thank God I had a choice. Each of us is blessed with the gift of choice when facing adverse situations.

I meditated often on James 1:2-3: *Consider it all joy, my brethren, when you encounter various trials, knowing that the testing of your faith produces endurance.* This was the biggest trial I had ever faced, and the Bible said I should be joyful during this time. In 1 Peter 4:12-13 it says in part that I should *rejoice in the midst of my fiery ordeals and trials.* This is a far cry from a natural response, but I made the choice to trust in God and be joyful nonetheless.

Furthermore, 1 Corinthians 2:14 says; *But a natural man does not accept the things of the Spirit of God, for they are foolishness to him, and he cannot understand them, because they are spiritually appraised.* I believe the natural response to my situation would be to wallow in the circumstances and ultimately succumb to them, but this is not what God wants anyone to do. God asks us all to call on Him in our time of need, and to *draw near with confidence to the throne of grace, so that we may receive mercy and find grace to help in time of need* (Hebrews 4:16). And we are constantly reminded to *walk by faith and not by sight* (2 Corinthians 5:7).

When we choose to completely trust God and His Word and are not moved away from that hope as a result of challenging circumstances, then God *will* respond because He loves us and because He honors His Word! Remember, *If you abide in Me, and My words abide in you, ask whatever you wish, and it will be done for you* (John 15:7).

No matter what issues might be getting you down, are you willing to come boldly to that same throne of grace where the Living God awaits your cry? He loves you and desires to have a wonderful relationship with you. We only need to humble ourselves and become like children in our hearts: *God is opposed to the proud, but gives grace to the humble* (James 4:6). My trust in God is a living testimony to an awesome miracle—God fulfilling His Word because I believed Him all along. I cannot express in words how truly blessed I am. Whoever trusts in the Lord will not be disappointed.

WHERE ARE THE DOCTORS?

Surprisingly, the last appointment with my oncologist was a week and a half after being discharged from the hospital and about the time I stopped taking the drug Cyclosporine. I was at his clinic for regular blood transfusions, of course, but that was based on *my* scheduling the appointment for the transfusions.

None of the specialists at the University of Minnesota made an attempt to follow up with me either. We spoke only once when I met with them in mid-May, and I expected to hear back from them by June 1, the time they had set for me to decide if I was comfortable in having the team at the U of M perform my bone marrow transplant.

I was not particularly eager for their call, but I found their lack of follow-up interesting, especially when a marrow transplant fetches $450,000 per procedure. On another occasion in June, I attempted to get an appointment with a different oncologist to obtain another opinion, but his office never got back to me. That, too, I found interesting and concluded that our meeting was simply not meant to be. I planned to cancel an appointment with a new oncologist at the Mayo Clinic that was scheduled for late August because I felt strongly that my miracle was going to arrive before then.

All along, my spirit showed me that I would be miraculously healed, without a bone marrow transplant. If I would have been contacted and told that a perfect marrow match had been found, I would have declined the procedure. I was that certain.

CHELATION STARTED

Although tin and aluminum were unlikely to have been related to the destruction of my bone marrow, I felt chelation would not only lower my high metal levels but would also promote a healthier state for my body.

LOSING IT FAST!

On July 23, the day after starting chelation, I received both a platelet and hemoglobin transfusion. Everything seemed fine until the morning of July 26 when I felt very tired and a bit lethargic. I asked my wife to drive me to my 2:00 p.m. appointment at Healing Center International (HCI). When we arrived, I did not feel well at all. Something was wrong.

Elaine Bonn, a prayer counselor and the founder of HCI, met us as we arrived and noticed immediately that I did not look well. She directed me to rest in one of the rooms until she and another prayer minister could come in and pray for me. I sat down in a chair and immediately fell asleep. They woke me ten minutes later.

Elaine asked me when I had received my last transfusion. I told her it was three days ago, and she asked if I prayed over the blood as I was receiving it. Although I had always prayed in the past when I received blood, I could not remember doing so this last time. Elaine began praying and instantly sensed something was wrong with the blood I received from the last transfusion. She thought that something spiritual in nature might have transferred with the blood.

While she shared this with me, I became more lethargic, very dizzy, and felt my veins grow cold. My physical state declined rapidly, and I had no idea why. I envisioned being rushed back to the hospital in an ambulance to get this blood out of me before it was too late. I felt like I would lose consciousness. I did all I could to maintain a state of awareness and not freak out. "Lord, help me!" I kept saying to myself. Elaine, knowing something was definitely wrong, took me back mentally to when I got the transfusion. She prayed for the blood as I received it, asking the Lord to make it pure with His blood and to filter anything not of Him from flowing into my body. She and the other prayer minister prayed for ten to fifteen minutes, and as they did, I began to feel better; my racing thoughts slowed. On the drive home, I gained more strength and clarity of mind. By evening, I was completely refreshed and felt wonderful.

Once again, God protected me! Whatever was going on with my body and blood that day, God intervened and turned a possible disaster into another miracle. I was truly at the right place at the right time that day!

CHELATION ABORTED

At the end of my visit to HCI on July 26, Elaine inquired about the chelation program I had started on July 22. We prayed about it, and Elaine felt led by the Lord to ask me to stop the program. Interestingly, when I began taking the chelation tablets, I was confused about the schedule. The more I studied about how I was supposed to take the tablets, the more questions I had, and the more confusing the schedule became. I took Elaine's suggestion as if it were the Lord's and aborted the chelation program that day.

BLOOD NUMBERS FALL, THEN RISE

My next blood test confirmed that chelation was not right for me. Just prior to beginning the chelation program, my percentage allocation of the white cells was within the normal range! The neutrophil percentage of white cells had risen to 45.2 percent (normal is 45 to 76 percent), and the lymphocyte percentage had dropped to 39.5 percent (normal is 15 to 43 percent)!

Once the chelation began, however, the percentages quickly reversed and fell out of the normal ranges. The white cell count also declined after I started the chelation program. The Lord spoke to Elaine while I was at the HCI and urged her to have me stop the chelation before the blood test results indicated that it was damaging to me. Without the Lord speaking to Elaine, I would have continued to take the chelation tablets, and my condition could have grown even worse. After stopping the chelation program, the declining white cell numbers reversed and began improving again. Those four days of chelation erased three to four weeks of white count progress.

AUGUST 15, 2001

A CURSE IS BROKEN!

On August 3, after a scheduled platelet transfusion, I headed to the northern Twin Cities suburb of Arden Hills to attend part of the annual Holy Spirit Conference held at North Heights Church. I was particularly interested in an afternoon session featuring a woman named Marlene who was scheduled to speak about how the Lord healed her twenty years earlier. She had suffered all her life with cerebral palsy and was miraculously healed by the Lord.

Her story was incredible, and I felt blessed to hear it. At the end of her talk, she handed the microphone to an elderly gentleman who invited anyone who wanted prayer for healing to come forward so that Marlene could pray for him or her. Half the room of over two hundred people went forward. I did not particularly feel drawn to ask for a healing prayer, but I asked God, "Do you want me to go forward and pray with Marlene?" I patiently waited for an answer. After a minute or two of silence, the Lord said no and prompted me to go and pray with the man (referring to the man who had invited people to pray with Marlene).

I immediately walked from the back of the room to this man who was packing his briefcase and preparing to leave. His handwritten name badge read John. I asked John if I could pray with him, and he said he would and asked me what I would like to pray about. I said that I was in the hospital back in April, that I was there for a month, and that the doctors diagnosed me with a blood disease they said was going to kill me.

"Stop!" he boldly interrupted. And, with an illuminated expression, he reached out, put his hand on my head, and said, "The Lord has these words for you: 'A curse has come against your bone marrow from four generations ago, and I'm breaking it now and filling your bones with fresh, clean, healthy marrow!'"

A curse has come against your bone marrow from four generations ago, and I'm breaking it now and filling your bones with fresh, clean, healthy marrow!

I could not believe what he said! We had not discussed the diagnosis or prognosis! I was amazed and shocked! I began laughing and crying at the same time and asked him how he knew that. He simply said the Lord had used him this way for years, and he walked out of the room.

I immediately called home to my wife and told her it was done and that my miracle had arrived in the physical! I began running around the church telling several of my friends that were at the conference: "It is done! My healing miracle has come! A curse has been broken! The manifestation has arrived!"

Marlene never spoke about generational curses; it was not the topic of the day at the conference. John (who I later learned was an evangelist living in Iowa) knew nothing about my condition, or me, yet he shared a word from the Lord about a generational curse and restoring my bone marrow! His prophetic words aligned with what the Lord told me on May 13 when He said He would *plant the seed of marrow and it would grow a hundredfold*. I believe a hundredfold meant *perfect* or *full*. And through John, God said He was filling my bones with marrow!

John's words, "fresh, clean, healthy marrow," were nearly identical to the very words I spoke out loud each day since I wrote them on a sticky note and stuck them on my wall at home! My note read; *Thank You, Father, for the fresh, powerful, and healthy bone marrow!* In addition, John's prophetic words confirmed Marjorie Cole's idea of a possible generational curse that needed to be broken. God chose to personally break it!

As these details unfolded I was simply amazed. Sometimes I cannot even believe it myself. It's almost beyond belief! But the most exciting part is that it is all true!

BLOOD NUMBERS—A CLOSE LOOK

On August 10, the white count inched again to a new high of 1,900! The average white count was 500 during the month of April, 925 in May, 1,250 in June, 1,683 in July, and 1,900 in August! With the normal range being between 3,500 10,800, I was more than halfway to normal!

The neutrophils reached 0.8 on August 10, which was also a new high. The average monthly counts were 0.0 in April, 0.15 in May, 0.385 in June, and 0.667 in July, and they were now at 0.8! With the normal range being between 1.9 and 8.0, I was now nearly one half of the way to a normal level!

We continued to see healthier white cell percentages. Unfortunately, the chelation program set my progress back about three to four weeks. After discontinuing the chelation, however, the allocation percentages of the three primary white cell types—neutrophils, lymphocytes, and monocytes—continued to improve.

The turnaround in the health of the white cell percentages after I began taking herbs and received the word from the Lord on May 13 were significant:

White Cell Percentages	May 10	July 12	August 10	Normal Range
Neutrophils	7.4%	41.0%	42.4%	45.0 – 76.0%
Lymphocytes	83.4%	44.1%	46.7%	15.0 – 43.0%
Monocytes	19.6%	13.4%	9.2%	0.0 – 10.0%

BLOOD NUMBERS

August 10	My Blood Counts	Notes	Normal Range
Red	10.4	Last Transfusion: 18 Days Ago	13.5 – 17.5
White	1,900	Count 11 Days Ago: 1,500	3,500 – 10,800
Platelets	26,000	Last Transfusion: 7 Days Ago	130,000 – 430,000
Neutrophils	0.8	Count 11 Days Ago: 0.6	1.9 – 8.0

August 10: The counts from my regularly scheduled blood tests are listed above. The white count and neutrophils improved ever so slightly but recovered nicely after being set back significantly by the chelation program. As of August 10, I had 179 tubes of blood drawn since the onset of illness. My vision continued to improve and was nearly normal.

CLOSING VERSES

. . . fixing your eyes on Jesus, the author and perfecter of faith . . .

(Hebrews 12:2)

Therefore, there is now no condemnation for those who are in Christ Jesus.

(Romans 8:1)

For I know the plans I have for you, says the Lord, plans for welfare and not for calamity to give you a future and a hope.

(Jeremiah 29:11)

How will we escape if we neglect so great a salvation?

(Hebrews 2:3)

AUGUST 26, 2001

MY STATEMENT SHOCKED HIM

On the afternoon of August 16, I had the first appointment in over ninety days with my primary oncologist—the one I saw daily while in the hospital. Even though the oncologist had been monitoring my test results, it was necessary to have an official appointment with him in order for me to continue receiving blood transfusions. Over the previous three months, I often felt written off as a patient, possibly due to the fact that I went against the doctors' recommendations and stopped taking Cyclosporine, or perhaps some had become nervous about the strong attitude of faith I maintained at a time when the doctors all seemed pessimistic about recovery.

Shortly after I arrived at the oncologist's office, I was brought into the examination room where the nurse asked me what medications I was taking. I chuckled inside thinking, *Shouldn't you know a bit more about your patient?* I replied, "No medications—none since May."

When the oncologist arrived and began looking over my steadily rising blood counts, I was hoping he would express some long awaited optimism. To the contrary, he said, "The numbers are improving some—they're certainly not going down."

I felt like saying *brilliant observation*, but, of course, I did not. I was simply hoping he would acknowledge that a miracle was in progress and be a little amazed by something he could not explain medically. He acknowledged there must be marrow present for these numbers to be rising to the levels they were. In an attempt to justify why the blood counts had risen, he admitted there must have been marrow all along and the treatment, which was deemed a failure back in April, must now be working suddenly in August! He seemed to be fighting to find an explanation. Knowing he was feeling uncomfortable, I did not challenge his opinions; I simply listened.

Throughout, the professional opinions remained the same: six doctors—including oncologists, surgeons, and pathologists from United Hospital and the University of Minnesota—all concluded there were no marrow stem cells present on April 9, when the biopsy was done. The neutrophil count was 0.0 all throughout April 2001, providing further evidence of the absence of bone marrow. The U of M team stated I had an "unfortunate case of bad luck." Each of these doctors concluded that death was the likely outcome since there was no marrow, no matching marrow donor, and the fact that marrow does not grow back.

The conversation with my oncologist continued with me asking, "What will it take . . ."

The doctor interrupted and completed my sentence: ". . . to make me happy?"

"Yes," I replied, with a smile.

The oncologist continued, "If your blood levels reached a point where you no longer needed *regular* transfusions, I'd be happy. Your levels will always be *less than normal*, but if they rise a bit more we could sustain you with periodic versus regular transfusions."

Knowing that he and I had totally different expectations, I asked, "What would prevent my blood levels from returning to normal?"

His response was, "With aplastic anemia, your blood levels will never return to normal. Furthermore, the disease can become aggressive at any time causing your levels to fall again."

With full assurance, I said, "Maybe so, but I don't have aplastic anemia any longer; it is gone, and it's not coming back!" I affirmed to him that my blood counts would rise to normal again. My statement shocked him, and then to my surprise, he asked if I wanted to return to the hospital and repeat the ATG treatment. I politely said, "No thank you."

It is interesting to note that this discussion with my oncologist was based upon the blood results from the previous week. Although I was not scheduled for a blood test until the following day, he suggested I have one taken while I was there. I agreed.

The test results were excellent, with platelets jumping to 46,000! As a result, I canceled my scheduled platelet transfusion for the following day but kept my appointment for the next blood test on August 23.

LIKE DEER IN THE HEADLIGHTS

After being released from the hospital, I frequently ran across various Christian doctors and nurses who were not involved in treating me. I shared my story with them, and a high percentage of them maintained the same viewpoint—*medical science is your only answer.* Surprisingly so, when I got to the faith, healing, and miracle portions of my story, nearly all became like deer caught in the headlights. They couldn't seem to grasp it—even those who said they have the faith!

The concept of supernatural healing has a tendency to challenge many, especially those in the medical field whose training is based on facts and science and not on faith and invisible attributes. Science strives to provide explanations, while miracles oftentimes cannot be explained. It's been pointed out to me by persons in the medical profession that God could heal me *through a bone marrow donor.* I typically responded by saying that I agree. Then I would always add, "But deep down in my spirit, I don't believe I will need a marrow transplant because God has shown me differently."

The common response back to me would be: "Well if your numbers fall back down, you would consider a transplant would you not?"

I again would have to clarify my position by saying, "They are not going to fall back; God is not going to do a halfway job. He is going to do a wonderful, miraculous job, just as His Word and Spirit have promised me." Right about there I would lose many, as my faith concept flew right over their heads.

I firmly believe that God *does* heal through medicine and through doctors, but *in my personal case,* I have come to believe something different occurred—a total supernatural healing! I believe each person should search their heart, listen closely for the answers to their prayers, and act accordingly. God promises that His Holy Spirit will lead us into all truth.

DANIEL'S TRIAL

God is the same yesterday, today, and forever. Many have heard the story of Daniel and the lion's den. The basics of the story go like this: Daniel was a faithful man who prayed openly three times a day. There were those who were jealous of Daniel and sought to destroy him by persuading the king to pass a law against prayer. They believed that Daniel would continue to pray anyway, thereby violating the king's decree. They would then force the king to uphold his law and put Daniel to death by feeding him to the lions. This is exactly what happened; Daniel was thrown into the lion's den.

Daniel trusted God for protection while he spent the night among the hungry lions. In the morning, the king commanded his guards to open the den and see whether Daniel's God had delivered him. Daniel was unharmed. The king ordered Daniel out and ordered Daniel's accusers thrown into the lion's den. Scripture reports that before Daniel's accusers even hit the ground, they were torn apart by the lions. Scripture tells us that God sent an angel to shut the mouths of the lions while Daniel was in the den. He was under God's care and protection because Daniel trusted God. God heard Daniel's prayer and honored his faith and his cry in his time of need. This is a miracle, an event that is difficult to explain with reason (see Daniel 6:1-28).

In the same way, under the care and power of the same God, the one that Daniel served thousands of years ago, I too called, trusted, and waited. With my being exposed to sick adults and children off and on during the time of a critically compromised immune system, God sent His angels (protection) to shut the mouth of a killer disease called aplastic anemia and also to protect me against any cold, flu, or other germs that could kill me. Is there any difference between these two miraculous outcomes other than the details? There isn't. They are both miracles. I serve the same God that Daniel served. God is no respecter of persons. He can do the same for you as He did for me, and as He did for Daniel: *And without faith it is impossible to please Him, for he that comes to God must believe that He is and that He is a rewarder of those who seek Him* (Hebrews 11:6).

LET THERE BE NEUTROPHILS!

During my appointment on August 16, the oncologist pointed out that the most important number he was watching was the neutrophil number (the primary indicator of the strength of the immune system.) He continued to remind me that any good news I might be reading into my numbers was irrelevant (i.e. the percentages of the various white cells within my immune system). "The neutrophils are everything," he'd say.

I could not agree more: "Let there be neutrophils!" On August 23, my neutrophil count had soared. It was double the count from just a week earlier, and this latest number of 2.0 placed my neutrophil count within the normal range! The total white count, the red count, and the platelets were all below normal but were rising! My oncologist was unavailable for comment.

THE DEVIL IS A LIAR

Even after all this great news, the devil loved to throw doubt and fear into my mind, especially on the way to the clinic each week to obtain my blood tests. He loved saying, "The best is behind you. Those good blood counts can't last. They'll be down today. No one survives this disease. It's not really marrow; it's just a bi-product of the transfusions you've received." But I simply chose not to listen to his lies. The Bible says; *Greater is He who is in you than he who is in the world* (1 John 4:4). We are to *resist the devil and he will flee from you* (James 4:7). Do you know something? It works! Therefore, *put on the full armor of God that you may be able to stand firm against the schemes of the devil* (Ephesians 6:11).

BLOOD NUMBERS

Blood Numbers	Aug 10	Aug 16	Aug 23	Normal Range
Red	10.4	10.4	10.6	13.5 – 17.5
White	1,900	2,100	3,000	3,500 – 10,800
Platelets	26,000	46,000	31,000	130,000- 430,000
Neutrophils	0.8	1.0	2.0	1.9 – 8.0

August 23: Red cells were last transfused on July 23, and platelets were last transfused on August 10. I was believing that I would ever need another blood transfusion! The neutrophils were now within the normal range! The white cells continued to climb and were nearing the normal range! My vision tested at 20/20! My weight remained steady.

White Blood Cell Percentages

White Cell Percentages	Aug 10	Aug 16	Aug 23	Normal Range
Neutrophils	42.4%	46.9%	67.3%	45.0 – 76.0%
Lymphocytes	46.7%	42.4%	25.4%	15.0 – 43.0%
Monocytes	9.2%	9.4%	7.3%	0.0 – 10.0%

The white cell percentages (allocation) of my immune system were now all within the normal range!

In Closing

I was reminded that the time was drawing near for me to deliver *the letter* that the Lord asked me to write on April 14 while in the hospital. I wrote it for the doctors and nurses who took care of me at the hospital and at the clinic. I was planning to share this letter with each of them when my blood levels reach normal as a testimony of having *perfect health in the presence of you all.*

Closing Verses

And there is salvation in no one else; for there is no other name under heaven that has been given among men by which we must be saved.

(Acts 4:12)

For I will restore you to health and I will heal you of your wounds, declares the LORD.

(Jeremiah 30:17)

How will we escape if we neglect so great a salvation?

(Hebrews 2:3)

SEPTEMBER 17, 2001

BLOOD NUMBERS WORSEN

Ever since the encouraging test results on August 23, I was very excited about the increasing blood numbers, especially the white counts (my immune system). The numbers, however, were not destined to stay there. The following week, on August 30, the white count fell from 3,000 to 2,600, and the neutrophils were no longer in the normal range, falling from 2.0 to 1.5. Both the hemoglobin and platelets counts remained fairly steady without the need of a transfusion, but what was happening to the white cells? Why were they falling? One week later, on September 6, I received more bad news—the blood numbers fell even further. The hemoglobin count sank to 10.1 from 11.0 a week earlier, representing the lowest level since my last red cell transfusion back on July 23. The last thing I wanted was another transfusion, especially now that I believed I would never need another one. The white cell count and neutrophils both plummeted, with the white count falling to 2,100 from 2600, and the neutrophils to 1.2 from 1.5. Just two weeks earlier, these numbers had been 3,000 and 2.0, respectively. I had no idea what was happening.

A HUGE TEST OF FAITH

The enemy immediately took advantage of these lower numbers and came in like the proverbial flood, bombarding me with fearful thoughts of more transfusions, a failed healing, an unbroken curse, and death. It was awful. So much progress had been made, and now it was being erased. This news seemed worse to me than the news of the initial diagnosis back in April! I was so excited and optimistic after experiencing the rising blood numbers over the previous weeks, and now I felt like I was heading back to square one.

After receiving these terrible blood results, I began to feel weaker, both physically and emotionally. A powerful negative effect had begun to take place. I felt spiritually disappointed. Was this truly an attack by the enemy to discourage me, or was it simply the hard cold facts? I then reminded myself, I MUST walk by faith and not by sight! These circumstances were trying to derail my faith! The devil was simply trying to steal, to kill, and to destroy! I could not be blind to his schemes! If I give up, I lose! I made the emotional and spiritual choice right then and there; I was *taking up the shield of faith with which you will be able to extinguish all the flaming arrows of the evil one* (Ephesians 6:16). And I stood on the same exact verses as I did from the beginning. This victory was mine and not the enemy's! It was not time for me to feel defeated or to become complacent; I needed to continue fighting this spiritual battle all the way through.

I began speaking out Biblical truths again: "Greater is He who is in me than he who is in the world; Jesus came to give life and to give it more abundantly; When the enemy comes in like a flood, the Spirit of the Lord will raise up a standard against him!" I prayed, got prayer, and confessed my healing out loud. My strength and faith increased. I was not going to allow the enemy to thwart the healing and incredible blessing that belonged to me! This was *my* victory! I was going all the way across the goal line to score that touchdown!

During these most challenging days, I was reminded of the passage in James once again; the one that has been my strength from the beginning of my battle: *Consider it all joy my brethren when you encounter various trials, knowing that the testing of your faith produces endurance* (James 1:2-3). I was simply being tested once again—this time more intensely than ever. I realized all those prior tests and trials had developed the endurance I now needed for strength so that I would not quit or be emotionally or spiritually overcome!

IMMUNE SYSTEM SOARS—REACHES NORMAL RANGE

The next week's visit to the clinic, on September 13, brought wonderful results—the best ever! What a turnaround! By confessing God's Word out loud and not dwelling on the poor numbers or circumstances from the previous week, the power of God was once again manifested through faith! It was absolutely amazing because it worked! The white count (immune system), which had been beaten down for two weeks straight, had soared to a new high and moved into the normal range! It jumped all the way from 2,100 to 3,500, and the neutrophil count jumped from 1.2 to 2.0! Not only did the white counts soar, but so did the hemoglobin and the platelets! The hemoglobin rose from 10.1 to 11.4, and the platelets jumped from 35,000 to 54,000! All of these increased without transfusions! Tears of joy filled my eyes as I shared this good news! Yes, yes, yes! Amen!

WEBSITE COMING

Once *all* the blood counts returned to normal, and I was described as being in perfect health, I intended to deliver the verse Acts 3:16 to the world. This was the verse the Lord gave me on April 11 while in the hospital. He told me, *This is the verse you will share with everyone on the day you're made whole.* I knew that day was rapidly approaching. I planned to use a website to boldly announce the miracle the Lord has done in my life. So I reserved the URL—a most fitting one indeed—www.Acts316.org.

BLOOD NUMBERS

Blood Numbers	Aug 30	Sept 6	Sept 13	Normal Range
Red	11.1	10.1	11.4	13.5 – 17.5
White	2,600	2,100	3,500	3,500 – 10,800
Platelets	33,000	35,000	54,000	130,000 - 430,000
Neutrophils	1.5	1.2	2.0	1.9 – 8.0

September 13: Red cells were last transfused on July 23 and platelets on August 10. After forty-one blood transfusions, I did not expect I would ever need another! The neutrophils were back within the normal range! The white cells also entered the normal range! Since the onset of the illness, 185 tubes of blood had been drawn for testing.

WHITE BLOOD CELL PERCENTAGES

White Cell Percentages	Aug 23	Aug 30	Sept 6	Sept 13	Normal Range
Neutrophils	67.3%	58.5%	59.0%	58.1%	45.0 – 76.0%
Lymphocytes	25.4%	33.2%	38.0%	33.3%	15.0 – 43.0%
Monocytes	7.3%	8.3%	3.0%	8.6%	0.0 – 10.0%

The white cell percentages (allocation) of my immune system were positioned well within the normal range!

CLOSING VERSES

[If] My people who are called by My name, humble themselves and pray and seek My face and turn from their wicked ways, then I will hear from heaven, will forgive their sin, and will heal their land.

(2 Chronicles 7:14)

Jesus said to him, 'I am the Way, the Truth and the Life; no one comes to the Father but through Me'.

(John 14:6)

So faith comes from hearing, and hearing by the word of Christ.

(Romans 10:17)

How will we escape if we neglect so great a salvation?

(Hebrews 2:3)

OCTOBER 4, 2001

We all need to encourage others when they are sick. One of the reasons I sent long emails to thousands was so others would be encouraged and blessed with God's truth, particularly His truth concerning healing, as I am a living example. You would be surprised how people react when you reach out to help. Don't take it for granted that they don't want *your* help; people do want help, especially if they are sick or in need. They will appreciate it more than you could ever imagine. Not only will you bless them, but you too will be blessed for taking the time to reach out. Remember, *Faith without works is dead* (see James 2:14-26).

THE DOORSTEP OF NORMAL

My blood counts had somewhat stabilized, just outside the gates of normal. They had been rising nicely, but now appeared to have stopped. This was something the oncologist reminded me of the last time I saw him: *When you have aplastic anemia, the blood counts never go back to normal.* For all practical purposes I was feeling normal, but my blood numbers still put me at risk.

RED CELLS

After retreating to a level of 10.1 the previous month, the weekly hemoglobin numbers were 11.4, 12.4, and 12.4, respectively. I cannot express how good the 12.4 level felt. Not only did I have more energy, but, more importantly, I had more oxygen going to my brain which enabled me to think more clearly and more quickly. For nearly five months, my low hemoglobin counts (between 7.5 and 10.5) affected the clarity and crispness of thought that I otherwise enjoyed at my pre-illness hemoglobin count of 15.4.

WHITE CELLS

Every third week we experienced the white counts jump upward to new highs followed by two weeks of lower numbers. I know that is not scientifically explainable, but this was the unique pattern that was recorded over the previous six week period: 3,000, 2,600, 2,100, 3,500, 3,200, and 3000.

Every time the numbers dropped, I would get barraged with thoughts from the enemy that I would be stuck with these low levels, that I would get sick again, or that the aplastic anemia was still there and could become "aggressive at any time," as the oncologist had told me. I realized this was nonsense—lies from the devil. The Bible tells us: *Resist him (the devil), firm in your faith* (1 Peter 5:9) and *Put on the full armor of God so that you will be able to stand firm against the schemes of the devil* (Ephesians 6:11). This is exactly what I chose to do through faithful affirmations!

PLATELETS

Likewise, the platelets followed an interesting pattern, although it was too early at this point to believe this specific pattern would continue. The platelets hung in a tight range of 31,000, 33,000, and 35,000. From there, they jumped to 54,000, 52,000, and 59,000. They were definitely getting better, and I expected them to keep climbing to perfect levels—above 130,000.

PRESS ON TO PERFECTION

It had become increasingly more comfortable to simply sit back and enjoy the life-sustaining blood numbers that I had. They were so much better than what I had been dealing with earlier in the year. Besides, it felt great not to have undergone a blood transfusion in nearly two months. Yet, at the same time, I had to avoid the tendency to thank the Lord for what He had done to this point and leave it at that since the Lord had been telling me something different all along—that I would be fully healed!

On four specific occasions, the Lord spoke to me about *full* restoration—to perfection! I believed that. I could not settle for acceptability but only for the fullness of the promise. The enemy would have had me bask in my partially restored health, even though it was not perfect. But God had a bigger plan, and somehow I was part of it. I was nearly over the goal line; the enemy was making his last stand, his last attempt to foil the promise of *perfection*. He would not prevail. The Lord was about to carry me over the goal line for that prized touchdown!

The *first* promise of perfection came on April 5, two days prior to being admitted to the hospital. It was 4:00 a.m. in the morning. I awoke coughing up blood and went downstairs for a snack. I turned on the television only to find a channel that had a Bible verse displayed on the screen. It was 1 Peter 5:10; this verse was for me, and God was telling me what was to come: *After you have suffered a little while, the God of all grace, who called you to His eternal glory in Christ, shall Himself, restore, strengthen, perfect, establish and confirm you.* I received this by faith that night, just as I hold firm to it today. I was restored and strengthened. I was soon to be perfected (with perfect blood numbers). I didn't know what the Lord planned to do to establish and confirm me, but I looked forward to it.

The *second* promise came on April 11, the fifth day in the hospital and the day after I was diagnosed with aplastic anemia. The Lord spoke again through His Word as I was reading Acts 3:16: *On the basis of faith in His name, it is the name of Jesus which has strengthened this man whom you see and know; and the faith which comes through Him has given him* [me] *this perfect health in the presence of you all.* This verse came alive in my spirit. I said, "This is me!" And the Lord instantly spoke to me saying, *This is the verse you will share with everyone on the day you're made whole.* ('Made whole' means made perfect!)

The *third* promise came on May 13, nine days after coming home from the hospital with no sign of marrow in my bones. As I was praying prior to going to bed, the Lord spoke to my spirit saying, *A farmer does not plant a seed in the field until he tills it, readies it, and then takes care of the field. You do likewise with your body, and I will plant the seed of marrow and it will grow a hundredfold.* Once again, God's words matched up with what He spoke through His Word in the first two promises. This time He was very specific and personal. God said He would plant the seed of marrow and that it would grow. In the parable of the sower (see Matthew 13:18-23), seed fell on the road, the rocks, the thorns, and the good soil. The seed that fell on the good soil was described as producing thirty, sixty, and a hundredfold. The good soil was me taking care of my body (the tilling), and the promise was the seed of marrow which the Lord promised to plant and that would grow a hundredfold—it would be perfect!

The *fourth* promise of perfection came on August 3, while at North Heights Church when John received a prophetic word from the Lord which said, *A curse has come against your bone marrow from four generations ago; I'm breaking it now, and filling your bones with fresh, clean, healthy marrow.* It is so awesome to see how God speaks to us and how His Word is flawless. It is not always easy to hear His voice. It can be difficult to listen and easy to doubt. As I look back at these four promises, it was not possible at the time to see how they would all come together in the way they did. I simply believed His Word and acted on what I heard from Him at the time. Only now, do I see how these promises all lined up: *For I am confident of this very thing, that He who began a good work in you* [me] *will perfect it until the day of Christ Jesus* (Philippians 1:6).

SPEAK IT INTO EXISTENCE

I have learned we have authority over many things as believers, including our body—especially when it pertains to sickness. I have noted, on several occasions, my blood levels rose when I spoke openly to the marrow, the immune system, and the blood cells. This is the prayer of authority that I prayed over my body:

In the name of Jesus, I speak to you marrow, my friend, ordained by the Lord God to sustain life in my body, to grow according to the

Word of the Lord, and to produce the fullness of hemoglobin, the fullness of platelets, the fullness of white cells, and the fullness of a healthy immune system! I speak to you hemoglobin, platelets, white cells, and immune system to grow to your fullness in accordance with your production from the marrow, to strengthen and protect my body to which the Lord has given abundant life. I rejoice in what the Lord has done, for He has squashed the plans of the enemy, which were to steal, to kill, and to destroy. For the Lord Jesus has come to give life and to give it abundantly, not halfway and not as an unfinished work, but as one that will bring about completion and perfection to that which He has started! Be all the glory to God our Father and to His Son, the Lord Jesus Christ, by whose stripes I am healed! Amen!

THE DOCTOR CALLED ME!

On September 25, my oncologist called me to say, "You're certainly doing very well." I can't express how much that meant coming from the doctor who had been so negative about my health for so long. During our ten-minute conversation, he suggested I have my blood tested every two weeks instead of every week. More importantly, I had the chance to share a couple things with him. I pointed out that my blood tests seemed to indicate that the percentages of my white cells persistently worsened while I was taking Cyclosporine, and when I stopped taking the drug, the white cell percentages began improving almost immediately. He said there was no correlation. I proceeded to share what the Lord told me about tilling the soil of my body and that He would plant the seed of marrow and it would grow a hundredfold. I told him that is the reason my blood counts were rising and that *grow* meant over time and that a *hundredfold* meant perfection. I expressed *that* was the reason I was convinced my counts would return all the way to normal. The oncologist was utterly speechless.

I then mentioned I bought him a book and would drop it off the next time I was at his clinic. I told him it was an excellent read, written by a medical doctor who described how he combined his faith with his medical knowledge to treat and heal his patients. He seemed very happy about it.

IMMUNE SYSTEM BEING TESTED

In early October I lost my voice to a bout with laryngitis! It appeared to be following the course of a viral strain that had hit many people in the Twin Cities area at this time. Six family members at my home suffered with the same viral bug. The symptoms started with a scratchy throat then proceeded to a loss of voice, followed by a cough. With the entire family sick, I was more susceptible and unable to keep free from catching this virus.

My white count was 3,000 (normal range is 3,500 to 10,800). The neutrophils were 2.0 (normal range is 1.9 to 8.0). So, from those numbers, one would assume I was able to successfully fight off the virus. I didn't really know if it would take longer to get over, but I was thankful my blood counts were at these levels and not at the levels of the previous months.

I didn't call the doctor because I believed this was a common cold and case of laryngitis. I didn't want to be given antibiotics unless it was absolutely necessary, and I believed my new immune system was up for the test.

NUTRITIONAL UPDATE

I continued taking Dr. Richard Schulze's SuperFood breakfast drink of herbs, vitamins, and minerals each morning. As much as possible, I adhered to eating foods and drinking liquids according to my blood type. I believe these actions had a positive impact on my body as I continued to *till the field*. Additionally, I began taking some basic nutritional supplements manufactured by Mannatech. These products are designed to enable/enhance cellular communication on eight cellular levels. The average American diet only engages cellular communication on approximately two levels, resulting in a weaker immune system.

BLOOD NUMBERS

Blood Numbers	Sept 13	Sept 20	Sept 28	Normal Range
Red	11.4	12.4	12.4	13.5 – 17.5
White	3,500	3,200	3,000	3,500 – 10,800
Platelets	54,000	52,000	59,000	130,000 - 430,000
Neutrophils	2.0	2.0	2.0	1.9 – 8.0

September 28: Red, white and platelet counts stabilized outside the normal ranges. Red cells were last transfused on July 23 and platelets on August 10. After forty-one blood transfusions, I did not expect I would ever need another! Since the onset of the illness, 187 tubes of blood had been drawn for testing.

WHITE BLOOD CELL PERCENTAGES

White Cell Percentages	Sept 13	Sept 20	Sept 28	Normal Range
Neutrophils	58.1%	61.0%	66.1%	45.0 – 76.0%
Lymphocytes	33.3%	32.0%	25.4%	15.0 – 43.0%
Monocytes	8.6%	7.0%	8.5%	0.0 – 10.0%

All these white cell percentages (allocation) were great. I will never forget when the neutrophils percentage was 7.4, and the lymphocyte percentage was 83.4. Then the herbs and a direct word from the Lord resulted in a 180-degree, miraculous turnaround. No treatment! No transplant! Just a miracle! What a journey!

CLOSING VERSES

... whosoever will call on the name of the Lord will be saved.

(Romans 10:13)

And we know that God causes all things to work together for good to those who love God, and to those who are called according to His purpose.

(Romans 8:28)

For there is one God, and one mediator also between God and men, the man Christ Jesus.

(1 Timothy 2:5)

How will we escape if we neglect so great a salvation?

(Hebrews 2:3)

OCTOBER 20, 2001

This is the day which the Lord has made. Let us rejoice and be glad in it! (Psalm 118:24)

I was so confident that my full, complete, and miraculous restoration to health would soon arrive. I was getting somewhat anxious to return to the doctors and nurses who took care of me while in the hospital and clinics to show myself as a perfectly healed man! I looked forward to handing each of them a copy of the letter I wrote back in April while in the hospital. Along with that letter, I wanted to provide them with a perfect CBC blood test to prove my perfect health as a testimony that God heals today!

I felt as if I could go today since I felt so great, but the numbers needed to be perfect for my visit to have the proper impact.

IMMUNE SYSTEM RESPONDS

The cold I caught in early October that resulted in laryngitis, expanded into my head and upper chest area. This particular strain of the common cold ran its course in just over a week. I heard from several others that they too battled this same viral strain—but for some it lasted for well over a month!

On the third day after the onset of this cold, I had a scheduled blood test at the clinic. My white count had risen to 6,000, exactly double from the previous week. The neutrophils more than doubled to a count of 4.1! This rapid increase in the numbers proved that once my body came under pressure, the marrow went to work and kicked out white cells to fight and kill off the cold virus! Most people would take this automatic response for granted, but having been without an immune system, I can assure you just how precious these increased numbers were.

I took no medication or antibiotics. My system worked efficiently and effectively all on its own. Because a cough developed and my chest became tight, I made two separate trips to the clinic to ensure that pneumonia was not developing. On both visits, the doctor indicated that my lungs sounded clear.

This type of viral cold could have killed me had I contracted it a month or two earlier. At that time, the extremely low white count not only made me highly susceptible to becoming sick, but it made fighting off any virus or bacteria virtually impossible. I'm so grateful. The Lord's protection every step of the way was nothing short of amazing.

HOW THE MARROW WORKS

Bone marrow is an amazing component of the human body. It represents the inner most part of human physiology. It is the factory that produces the three major blood components that are essential for life.

In an attempt to understand why my platelet and hemoglobin counts stabilized below the normal levels, I needed to understand more about how the marrow worked—and I did quite a bit of personal research on the topic. Marrow works in response to the demand, or tax, on the body. When white cells are needed to fight a foreign invader, the marrow produces more white cells. When platelets are needed to repair a cut or bruise, the marrow produces more platelets. Likewise, when hemoglobin is needed to supply more oxygen to the body, the marrow produces more hemoglobin.

Since the Lord had planted fresh, healthy marrow back in my bones, my body had only had one fire call—the viral cold I experienced. This event caused the marrow to do its job perfectly, by producing the increase in white cells! On the other hand, there had not been a tax on my body with respect to a cut or bruise (platelets) or a call for additional oxygen (hemoglobin). As a result, my body had not told the marrow to produce more than what is necessary. This was my hunch as to why my levels had stopped rising and stabilized a bit short of normal ranges. Now, I needed to confirm my hunch by performing a little test.

MY PART—HIS PART

I thought I had already done all the right stuff, but I began to sense that I was missing a very important component of this process of healing. I was eating properly, getting plenty of rest, but I was not exercising. Exercise, of course! This made perfect sense. If I were to exercise, I would be taxing my body and putting a demand on my marrow to produce more hemoglobin to carry the needed oxygen to my muscles and organs.

I was anxious to run this idea past any of the doctors at the clinic. On my next visit, I asked a doctor whether exercise would increase the hemoglobin levels in my blood. After acting surprised that I was not exercising, he went on to say that exercise would not only increase my hemoglobin levels but also increase my platelet levels. I felt like informing this doctor how I was previously instructed not to exercise but felt it did not matter now. What I just heard was awesome news. There it was: the missing component!

Then this dawned on me: What have we heard since childhood? To be healthy we need to eat right, get plenty of rest, and exercise regularly. This is exactly what the Lord was saying when He said; *Take care of your body like the farmer takes care of the field . . .* In other words, *You do the part that only you can do, and I will do the part that only I can do!*

AT THE YMCA!

Still enthused by what the doctor said about exercise being able to boost my stagnant blood levels, I went down and purchased a family membership at the YMCA. I went regularly for about a week, and I cannot tell you how out of shape my muscles had become, not having exercised at all that year. My body had felt fine sitting in a chair at the office, talking on the phone or getting in and out of the car, but lifting weights and jogging again—wow! My body was definitely being taxed.

I eventually managed to jog one mile without stopping! This was a great accomplishment for me, even though it took over 9 minutes. I planned to gradually increase the frequency and intensity of the workouts. It was painful, but I needed to press on and push my blood levels to normal. Simply telling the doctors and nurses I had been healed would not work—they would not believe me. The *only* thing they would believe would be the blood numbers.

BLOOD NUMBERS

Blood Numbers	Sept 20	Sept 28	Oct 5	Oct 12	Normal Range
Red	12.4	12.4	12.4	12.2	13.5 – 17.5
White	3,200	3,000	6,000	4,500	3,500 – 10,800
Platelets	52,000	59,000	56,000	65,000	130,000 - 430,000
Neutrophils	2.0	2.0	4.1	3.4	1.9 – 8.0

October 12: White cells jumped as a result of the viral cold and were holding within the normal range. Red and platelet counts had stabilized outside the normal ranges. Red cells were last transfused on July 23 and platelets on August 10—for a total of forty-one transfusions. Since the onset of the illness, 189 tubes of blood have been drawn for testing.

WHITE BLOOD CELL PERCENTAGES

White Cell Percentages	Sept 20	Sept 28	Oct 5	Oct 12	Normal Range
Neutrophils	61.0%	66.1%	68.0%	75.7%	45.0 – 76.0%
Lymphocytes	32.0%	25.4%	28.0%	17.2%	15.0 – 43.0%
Monocytes	7.0%	8.5%	4.0%	7.1%	0.0 – 10.0%

All the percentages (allocation) of my primary white cells were in the normal range, with the neutrophils on the high end of normal as they increased to fight the viral cold.

CLOSING VERSES

For God so loved the world, that He gave His only begotten Son, that whoever believes in Him shall not perish, but have eternal life.

(John 3:16)

Jesus said to her, 'I am the resurrection and the life; he who believes in Me shall live even if he dies.'

(John 11:25)

How will we escape if we neglect so great a salvation?

(Hebrews 2:3)

NOVEMBER 21, 2001

HUNCH WAS CORRECT – BLOOD LEVELS SOAR!

My white blood count had doubled as a result of my body needing to fight off the cold virus. When my body was being tested, the new marrow proved to work just fine. My platelet and hemoglobin counts, however, had stopped rising and stabilized below normal levels. I had a hunch that my marrow would produce higher levels of platelets and hemoglobin as a result of exercise. My hunch was correct!

By moderately exercising a few times per week, I saw a dramatic rise in the hemoglobin count! The count, which had stabilized around 12.2, jumped to 13.9 after two weeks of exercise and then to 14.2 after another two weeks. The normal range for an adult male is 13.5 to 17.5, meaning my hemoglobin had reached normal! Three months prior, I could not jog a single block due to excruciating pain in my legs from the lack of oxygen available to my muscles. Now, I was able to run a mile – in just 6:40!

Now, I was able to run a mile
– in just 6:40!

Likewise, the platelets began moving upward as a result of the exercise. They rose from 65,000 to 80,000 over a four-week period. I fully expected them to continue to rise to the normal range of 130,000 to 430,000. They were at their highest level since the marrow was destroyed back in April.

I still recall some of the interesting comments my oncologist made during our August 16 appointment: "When you have aplastic anemia, you will need a bone marrow transplant to rid yourself of the disease; otherwise, you will always have the disease and your blood numbers will never go back to normal."

My response to him was, "I don't have it anymore; I have been healed, and my numbers are going back to normal!" On that day, when I spoke those words to him, my hemoglobin was 10.4, my white count was 1,900, and my platelet count was 26,000. Now, those numbers had risen to 14.2, 5,200, and 80,000, respectively!

Although I had not spoken to my oncologist since late September, he had to be amazed at my blood tests. I know he saw them because each test result was faxed to his clinic in St. Paul. The counts kept increasing—how could he explain that? I knew he couldn't. That might be the reason I didn't hear from him. I still wonder if he ever asked himself, *Who is this faith-filled guy who says, 'I don't have it anymore; I have been healed, and my numbers are going back to normal?'*

AN ONSLAUGHT OF FEAR
It's quite amazing how the enemy constantly seeks ways to attack our thinking. He looks for any weak spot or circumstance to make

inroads into our lives—with one purpose: to steal, kill, and destroy. The devil used five circumstances as weapons to mount an all-out attack on me, but in the end I was able to maintain victory over him. The attack had been mounting, but on a particular Monday evening I was hit full force with his many weapons.

Circumstance one: On a Friday evening, I received a call from a person in my small group who informed me that his close friend was not expected to live through the night. This friend had been battling aplastic anemia as well and was about to be overcome by it. He had been doing very well, and his blood numbers were rising nicely. Then suddenly his white blood counts plummeted, he developed pneumonia, and he had been unable to fight it off. On Sunday, I learned from my small group friend that this person died over the weekend.

Circumstance two: During this same time, I ran across a neighbor who happened to be in the medical field. I had previous discussions with him about my health, faith, and miraculous progress. And even though I presented a convincing case, he remained somewhat skeptical. This day was no different. After I mentioned that all my blood levels were rising, he stated that "the hemoglobin and platelets really don't matter, because it is the white count that is most critical to health and that is usually what falls and causes those with aplastic anemia to die." This is exactly how the man in circumstance one died.

Circumstance three: After my bout with a cold in October, my white count dropped back down to 3,000 after rising to 6,000. I was not only discouraged that the count had fallen all the way down to 3,000, but it was no longer in the normal range. The enemy continued to bombard me with fearful thoughts that my white count would fall to dangerously low levels again, at any time and without warning.

Circumstance four: I had been watching and waiting for a small scar on my body to heal while these other things were transpiring. Instead of healing in five to seven days (what I would consider normal), it did not heal in over two weeks. Did the white count of 3,000 result in the scar taking longer to heal? Possibly. As minor as this may seem, it was just another issue that the enemy was using as he launched his assault, prompting me to think my white count was not good enough to keep me healthy and that I was not truly healed.

Circumstance five: The following Monday, I began to develop a runny nose and a very raspy throat. By the time evening arrived, I was finding it harder and harder to swallow. I realized it was the onset of a nasty cold. By bedtime, I had become physically uncomfortable. I felt terrible. More importantly, however, I was extremely discouraged that I was being hit by another cold as I had just got over one a few weeks earlier. This too became a weapon of the enemy—taunting me that my immune system could not even protect me from getting another cold. I tried to sleep but could not.

The assault mounted! The devil was throwing every spiritual weapon of fear and doubt at me. Those little voices in my mind would not let up, as they hammered and hammered on me: "There is no cure for aplastic anemia!" "Didn't the doctors tell you that!" "You're going to die, just like that person last Friday night!" "Your immune system is not working!" "Your nose is running from an infection in your throat." "Your white counts are falling and that's why that little scar won't heal!" "It's not a cold; you have pneumonia!" "Your body cannot fight it; it's too weak!" "The signs are clear all around you—why don't you accept it?" "Give up; you've lost the battle!" "You're going to die!"

Just before midnight, my wife and I prayed for protection from all these lies and negative thoughts. I tried to sleep, but the attack continued and began to escalate. I countered by speaking Scripture verses out loud, over and over again—knowing the sword of the

Spirit is the Word of God. I found myself in the midst of a major fight, a spiritual battle that went on and on. I would not succumb to fear, however! I stood my ground and continued speaking verses from God's Word out loud and then concluded by saying, "Greater is He who is in me than *you* who are in the world. Satan, you're the loser; you have lost this battle from the beginning, and you're even more of a loser because you don't see it. Take your lies and leave in Jesus' name!"

I remember this battle going on until 3:30 a.m., at which time I was finally able to sleep. I had never experienced anything like this; it was so intense. One thing had changed when I awoke a few hours later; the onslaught of fear that tried to overpower me had subsided, and the attack was over. Victory was mine! Even now, it is hard to explain it all. I can say this for sure: Satan used a number of specific and related circumstances and threw them at me like flaming missiles, one after another for hours while I was tired, weak, and wanting to sleep. Perhaps that was part of the enemy's goal line defense that I needed to break through in order to score my touchdown. I never had an attack of fear like that while in the hospital, but the victory was mine in the end through the Word of God! Yes, the Word of God; it *is* the Sword of the Spirit!

ANOTHER COLD PUT TO REST
This second cold did not last as long as the previous one. Its symptoms lasted just five days. Whether it was a weaker viral strain than the one I dealt with a few weeks earlier or whether my immune system simply worked better and quicker, I really don't know. Since I had a choice, I chose to believe the latter—that my immune system was better than ever.

GROUP TESTIMONY
I was blessed on November 18 to be able to share some of the miraculous details of what the Lord had done in front of a group of over 500 at Hosanna Church, where I attend services in Lakeville,

Minnesota. This was the first time I had the opportunity to give this marvelous testimony in front of a large group.

BLOOD NUMBERS

Blood Numbers	Oct 5	Oct 12	Oct 26	Nov 9	Normal Range
Red	12.4	12.2	13.9	14.2	13.5 – 17.5
White	6,000	4,500	3,000	5,200	3,500 – 10,800
Platelets	56,000	65,000	75,000	80,000	130,000 - 430,000
Neutrophils	4.1	3.4	1.7	3.5	1.9 – 8.0

November 9: White cells rose in response to both encounters with viral colds. Red and platelet counts increased in response to exercise. During the battle for my life, I had provided 191 tubes of blood for testing.

WHITE BLOOD CELL PERCENTAGES

White Cell Percentages	Oct 5	Oct 12	Oct 26	Nov 9	Normal Range
Neutrophils	68.0%	75.7%	56.0%	68.0%	45.0 – 76.0%
Lymphocytes	28.0%	17.2%	31.0%	23.0%	15.0 – 43.0%
Monocytes	4.0%	7.1%	9.0%	2.0%	0.0 – 10.0%

All the percentages (allocation) of my primary white cells were in the normal range, with the neutrophils on the high end of normal as they increased to fight the viral colds.

CLOSING VERSES

. . . God is opposed to the proud, but gives grace to the humble. Submit therefore to God . . . Resist the devil and he will flee from you. Draw near to God and He will draw near to you . . . Humble yourselves in the presence of the Lord, and He will exalt you.

(James 4:6-10)

You search the Scriptures, because you think that in them you have eternal life; it is these that testify about Me; and you are unwilling to come to Me so that you may have life.

(John 5:39-40)

Trust in the Lord with all your heart and do not lean on your own understanding. In all your ways acknowledge Him, and He will make your paths straight.

(Proverbs 3:5-6)

How will we escape if we neglect so great a salvation?

(Hebrews 2:3)

DECEMBER 12, 2001

The year 2001 will go down as a spectacular year, perhaps the best year of my life! Even though it began with a long string of unfortunate circumstances that never seemed to end, looking back now, it is clear to see why I needed those experiences. Not only was my faith being tested, but my spiritual strength was also being built up so that I had the endurance to get through the most challenging battle ever—the one for my life!

During the course of 2001, I learned more about blood, health, herbs, and healing than I could have ever imagined. There were thousands, most of whom I have never met, who gave me additional strength to forge ahead in my darkest hour. Yes, the Lord my God performed the miracle. He gave me the ultimate strength I needed and built me up when I was down, but many were there for me each step of the way with letters, cards, and emails that always showed support, concern, and love. Every time I learned that someone loved getting my emails, they were praying for me, or they had added me to a prayer chain, it touched my heart, fueled me, and empowered me to cross over that goal line. Even though I was the one carrying the ball, the one who scored this time, I feel that it was a team effort.

Never forget the significance of encouragement. The impact it can have in another person's life is incredible. A kind word here and a supportive comment there will inspire others to reach beyond all their preconceived limitations. Believing in others and making sure they know you believe in them matters. It truly does; I am living proof of that.

THE LETTER WAS DELIVERED!

As a result of my platelet counts soaring to 110,000 on December 7 and my white and hemoglobin counts well within the normal ranges, I felt this was the time to deliver the letter and show myself to the doctors and nurses as the restored and strengthened man who had been granted my Acts 3:16 destiny, having *this perfect health in the presence of you all!*

I waited a long time to deliver the letter that I wrote in the late hours of the night on April 14, 2001. The one entitled: *I've Been Miraculously Healed!* The fact that the letter was written immediately after receiving the dismal diagnosis and prognosis gave it greater significance.

I've Been Miraculously Healed!

On December 10, with a stack of the letters in hand, I made my way to United Hospital. I experienced the most incredible emotions as I walked into the oncology ward. Before speaking with anyone, I walked past the nurses' station and toward Room 4526, the room that had been my home for much of the month of April. I stopped outside the door to the room and, *in my mind*, briefly returned to this most interesting chapter in my life.

I saw the layout of the room and in it the faces of many visitors. I saw all the get well cards and balloons that lined the ledge in front of the window. In the bathroom, next to the sink was my feather-like toothbrush carefully sitting in the disinfected cup. I saw the walk-in shower that I waddled into each day as I pulled that silly apparatus-on-wheels alongside of me. It had held the bags of blood, saline, and antibiotics that were connected to my right arm through needles and IVs twenty-four hours a day. I remembered wrapping my arm each day in cellophane before making my way to the shower in order to protect all those needles. I saw the bed, the night lights and the ink marker board with all my Bible verses on it. How could I forget the blood cart alongside my bed and the oncologist delivering my diagnosis? I saw it quite vividly. I even caught a glimpse of myself doing a market evaluation on my laptop while sitting up in bed.

All this took just a few seconds, but the memories will last a lifetime. I realized then, more than ever, just how blessed I was not to be in that room any longer and that I was, in fact, a walking miracle.

I returned to the nurses' station where five nurses were hard at work. I recognized two of them as having cared for me earlier in the year. At first they did not recognize me, being they had not seen me since early May. After informing them of who I was, they responded, "Oh my gosh! You look great! So you got a bone marrow transplant?"

"No, I did not" I replied, "You do remember me saying the Lord was going to heal me miraculously don't you? Well, He did! No transplant! No medical explanation!" The nurses were amazed and puzzled at the same time but shared in my excitement. I began to share about the letter I had for them and how I had written it back in April from Room 4526. At this point, several of the nurses looked a bit shocked and weren't sure what to say. I left them copies of the letter and asked them to circulate it among the staff, the patients, and especially the doctors. They agreed.

I had really hoped to see my doctor, the oncologist who cared for me while I was at United. My last visit with him face-to-face was on August 16. I knew it would be good for him to see me, but it was not meant to be. As promised, I left him the book *Healing Prayer* by Dr. Reginald Cherry, M.D.

From the hospital, I headed to the clinic where I had been an outpatient for over three months. It was there that I had received all my blood transfusions after being sent home from the hospital. In like fashion, I visited with a couple of the nurses that had cared for me. They, too, were surprised, even thrilled. After visiting for at least an hour, I once again left a large stack of letters as a testimony of the miracle that God had performed in me.

A FINAL WORD

Before beginning my email communication, the Lord told me to tell *everyone... everything.* I was told to open up and share the detailed events as they happened, as well as describe certain events that had not yet occurred. I feel I have done that.

At the time I began writing, the Lord spoke something very profound to me. In fact, those words are more profound today than they were back then; they consistently bring joy to my heart and tears to my eyes: *I am going to show Myself strong through you before the eyes of many people.*

I am going to show Myself strong through you before the eyes of many people.

CHAPTER 5

— Restoration and New Life —

CHAPTER 5

As I look back over those critical months of being extremely ill, I appreciate the significance of recognizing those very special messages the Lord gave me—the promises of being healed. He always gave me just what I needed at the time I needed it so that I remained strong no matter what the circumstances.

BUSINESS RESTORED

While going through the challenges of 2001, the Lord also provided financially for me and my family. We actually did more real estate business while I was in the hospital and over the few months that followed than the last half of 2000! As I walked out on that branch of faith, going on listing appointments without an immune system, God continued to bless us with fruit from that labor.

The latter half of 2001 yielded a harvest of business. Sales began to roll in one after the other. The Lord restored the finances that were lost in 2000, and then some. When I was going through my tsunami of challenges, there was a moment of time when I compared myself to Job. I feel like the Lord restored me much like the actual story of Job. In February of 2002, RE/MAX North Central honored me with the *Spirit Award*, given to honor me for not only finishing 2001 as the second highest producing sales agent in Minnesota but also for the conditions under which those results were accomplished.

David Linger, the regional director, put it this way: "This award is not just an award about 'sales' but about 'attitude'—an attitude of faith, determination, and spirit. And, in this special case, an attitude that has resulted in a miraculous recovery from an incurable situation."

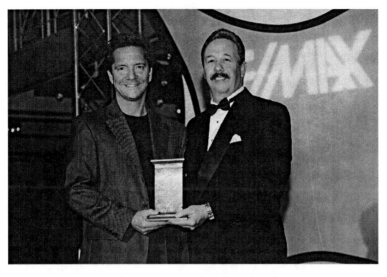

PRESENTATION OF THE 2001 "SPIRIT AWARD" BY RE/MAX
REGIONAL DIRECTOR, DAVID LINGER—FEBRUARY, 2002,
AT THE RE/MAX REGIONAL
AWARDS BANQUET IN MINNEAPOLIS, MINNESOTA

Real estate continues to be a blessing for my family and me. In 2004 I received the coveted Circle of Legends award, being one of only thirty-five sales associates among over 100,000 RE/MAX agents worldwide to have earned it in their careers. In 2006 I completed 283 sales transactions and placed first in sales in Minnesota and tenth in the United States. And in 2010 I was named National Marketer of the Year as the result of winning a competition that was open to real estate agents from across the nation.

MINISTRY

Since being healed there have been many opportunities to share about the goodness of God. Teaching classes designed to strengthen believers in their faith, challenging them to utilize their gifts and talents, and expressing in written form how God heals today are just a few of the ministry opportunities I have found. In addition,

I've traveled to several foreign countries on mission trips where I share this *Journey to a Miracle* testimony. *The Promise* – which is a short story where I encourage people to choose faith over fear when facing a major life crisis – is now in multiple languages.

WHO WAS THAT MAN NAMED JOHN?

Often, I am asked about the evangelist who prayed for me and the breaking of the generational curse over me and my bone marrow. I actually did not know who he was for over three years after our encounter on August 3, 2001, at North Heights Church. One day I got a tip on who he might be, and I followed up on it. I learned that his name was John Kittleson and that he lived in a small town in Iowa. I found his phone number, called him, and left him a message. When John called me back later that day, I reminded him of what had taken place on that very special day in August, and the amazing results that followed. After hearing the outcome, John stated that my healing was one of the top three miracles the Lord had worked through him. When I asked him about some of the others, he commented that the Lord once used him to raise up a man who had been dead for several minutes!

John Kittleson and I have spoken together at several ministry events and healing services where we taught and prayed for those that were in need of healing. John is an amazing man and has served as an evangelist for many years. According to John's own words, my healing was a most remarkable miracle: *I've been involved in the 'healing and deliverance' ministry for over thirty years. During this time, I have witnessed Jesus' miraculous touch many times. One of the most remarkable miracles that God has done was the deliverance and healing of Jeff Scislow from a fatal bone marrow disease. The Holy Spirit gave me a supernatural revelation of Jeff's condition, and I simply obeyed by breaking a genetic curse and commanding the disease to leave in Jesus' name and asking the Lord to give Jeff new bone marrow. The Lord honored Jeff's faith and ministry and healed Jeff. All the glory and praise to Jesus, the Healer!*

INSPIRATION TO FINISH THE FIRST DRAFT OF THIS BOOK

During the last week of January 2008, I traveled to Hawaii where I was speaking at an annual real estate event. I arrived a day early in order to spend time finishing what would be the first draft of this book. While in my hotel room, which overlooked the ocean, I opened up my balcony door to the fresh air and the sound of the waves below. As I began to write some of my final thoughts, a beautiful white dove landed on the railing of my balcony. It watched me as I worked for a moment. Then it hopped down onto the balcony floor, walked into my room, and stood in front of me. I reached for my camera to take a picture, expecting the flash to scare it off. It did not! In fact, I continued to take flash photos of the dove as it watched me and walked around my hotel room! It stayed with me for over thirty minutes before making its way back to the balcony and finally flying off again.

I am not certain whether this was a sign from God, but it was very inspiring to say the least—not only to me but also to those I have shared the story and photos with. For me, it was as if God inspired me to finish those last parts of the book and showed His approval by sending a dove.

DOVE PHOTOS

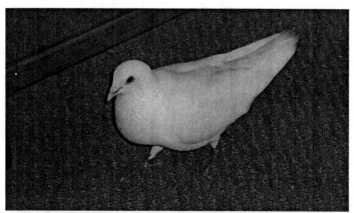

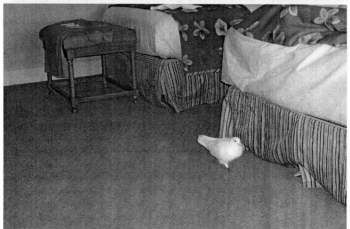

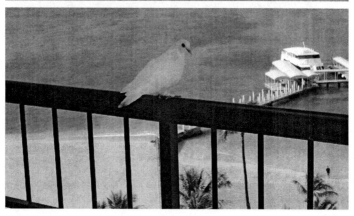

FOLLOW-UP VISITS

During 2002 I made eight bi-weekly visits to my local clinic for the purpose of follow-up blood testing; I decided to discontinue them after my eighth appointment since my blood counts during this period of time were quite good. In October 2003, I had an annual physical that included the standard blood tests—my counts were strong, and all other aspects of my health were excellent. In December 2004, I had another physical which again indicated a clean bill of health, and my platelets had *finally* risen above 130,000 and into the "normal" range! In December 2007, I went in for my next physical and once again, my blood counts were all normal.

To my amazement, I have not seen my oncologist once since my last face-to-face with him on August 16, 2001, nor have I spoken with him since late September 2001, when we talked on the phone. I have made several attempts to catch him at his clinic with no success. I even left him my testimony on CD in June 2002, and I also left him a business article on my success in the real estate industry in the fall of 2007. I have yet to hear from him. On a positive note, I have visited with several other doctors who work in the local clinics near my home. They have been supportive and certainly surprised and enthused by the miraculous outcome I have had the joy of experiencing.

DECEMBER 26, 2007, BLOOD TEST RESULTS

Order CBC W/ PLATELETES, DIFF [85025] Order #: 25851522 Spec #: W58662 Class: Normal

Patient Name	**Sex**	**DOB**
Scislow, Jeffrey Floyd	Male	
(0000018953)		

Results   CBC WITH PLATELETS, DIFF

Result Information

Result Date and Time	Status	Provider Status
12/26/2007 4:04 PM	In process	Ordered

Component Results

Component	Value	Flag	Low	High	Units	Stat
WBC	5.3		4.0	11.0	10e9/L	Fin
RBC	4.47		4.4	5.9	10e12/L	Fin
HGB	15.5		13.3	17.7	g/dL	Fin
Hct	43.6		40.0	53.0	%	Fin
MCV	98		78	100	fl	Fin
MCH	34.7	H	26.5	33.0	pg	Fin
MCHC	35.6		31.5	36.5	g/dL	Fin
RDW	12.7		10.0	15.0	%	Fin
PLT	209		150	450	10e9/L	Fin
Diff Method	Pending					Inc

These excellent blood results show the white cells at 5,300; hemoglobin at 15.5; and platelets at 209,000!

DAILY NUTRITION

I still take Dr. Richard Schulze's Superfood breakfast drink of herbs, vitamins, and minerals daily, and ever since 2001, I have subscribed to the advice of Dr. Peter D'Adamo's book *Live Right 4 Your Type*. I also use a wide variety of the excellent Melaleuca supplements and health products daily. I keep an open mind and continue to learn. In my experience, it is much easier to remain healthy by taking care of my body with a proper diet, restful sleep, and exercise, than it is to nurse it back to health were I to get sick.

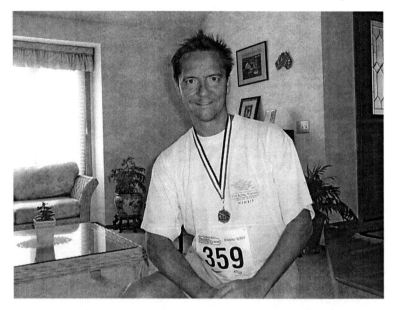

I STILL TRAIN AND RUN IN RACES PERIODICALLY, AND IN 2002 WAS A TOP FINISHER IN A LOCAL TWO MILE RUN.

MAKE THE MOST OF YOUR LIFE

My hope is that my story encourages others to make the most of their life, health, and relationships. Most of all, I pray that it encourages others to strengthen their relationship with God the Father, through His Son Jesus Christ. Without *that* relationship in place, nothing else matters at the end of the day. His love for each of His children is no different than His love for me, as He is not a respecter of persons. He plays no favorites. Jesus is the same yesterday, today, and forever. If you abide in Him and His words abide in you then you can ask anything, and He will do it for you. He is the Way, the Truth, and the Life; no one comes to the Father, but through Him.

CHAPTER 6

— Secrets of Healing —

Chapter 6

Most likely you know a friend or loved one who is currently battling a disease or illness; this may even describe you. In the course of my journey, I learned some crucial principles—that I like to call *secrets*—that paved the way for healing to take place. I firmly believe God is able and willing to heal *today*, but there are *hindrances* that can prevent us from receiving God's full plan for healing. The Bible is filled with conditions—with IFs and THENs— that illustrate when we do our part, God will do His part. Allow me to point out some of these and to share the secrets of healing that were part of my experience.

A Foundational Fact

Our battle is not against flesh and blood but against powerful rulers of darkness in the spiritual realm (see Ephesians 6:12). The devil and his angels are quite real and have a clear mission—one of deception, destruction, and death. We are instructed to take up the full armor of God (His truth, His Word, and our faith) to be able to withstand the fiery attacks of our spiritual enemy (see Ephesians 6:13-17). When we do this, we have armed ourselves for victory over the enemy, as evidenced in 2 Corinthians 10:4: *for the weapons of our warfare are not of the flesh, but divinely powerful for the destruction of (demonic) fortresses.* Our faith in God's promises is described as . . . *the victory that has overcome the world . . .* (1 John 5:4).

Source of Freedom and Healing

Jesus provides freedom, life, and victory over anything the devil throws at us, including sickness. He clearly tells us; *The thief* [the devil] *comes only to steal and kill and destroy; I came that they may have life, and have it abundantly* (John 10:10). Jesus is our source for healing: . . . *by His wounds you were healed* (1 Peter 2:24) and our source for freedom: . . . *if the Son makes you free, you will be free indeed* (John 8:36).

OBEDIENCE

Obedience is an important part of healing as well as a condition to getting prayers answered. Do not expect God to bless you if you are living in or practicing sin: . . . *your iniquities have made a separation between you and your God, and your sins have hidden His face from you so that He does not hear* (Isaiah 59:2). And from Proverbs we are told that; *He who turns his ear away from listening to the law* [God's Word], *even his prayer is an abomination* (Proverbs 28:9). But when we follow God's Word in obedience, the opposite is true, and we receive everything we ask from Him: *and whatever we ask we receive from Him, because we keep His commandments and do the things that are pleasing in His sight* (1 John 3:22).

The following verses from the Old Testament carry the same principle of obedience as a prerequisite to staying healthy and/or being healed: *And He said, 'If you will give earnest heed to the voice of the Lord your God, and do what is right in His sight, and give ear to His commandments, and keep all His statutes, I will put none of the diseases on you which I have put on the Egyptians; for I, the Lord, am your healer'* (Exodus 15:26); . . . *fear the Lord and turn away from evil, it will be healing to your body and refreshment to your bones* (Proverbs 3:7-8).

UNCONFESSED SIN

If your heart is revealing sin that needs to be confessed then confess—it is a prerequisite to having your prayers answered. God wants us to confess our sins to Him: *If we confess our sins, He is faithful and righteous to forgive us our sins and to cleanse us from all unrighteousness* (1 John 1:9). We are also instructed to: . . . *confess your sins to one another, and pray for one another so that you may be healed. The effective prayer of a righteous man can accomplish much* (James 5:16). King David made it quite clear in Psalm 66:18 that harboring sin prevents the Lord from hearing our prayers: *If I regard wickedness in my heart, the Lord will not hear.*

AN UNHARMONIOUS RELATIONSHIP

An unharmonious relationship between a husband and a wife will hinder prayer: *You husbands in the same way, live with your wives in an understanding way, as with someone weaker, since she is a woman; and show her honor as a fellow heir of the grace of life, so that your prayers will not be hindered* (1 Peter 3:7).

SELFISHNESS

Selfishness is another hindrance to prayer: *You ask and do not receive, because you ask with wrong motives, so that you may spend it on your pleasures* (James 4:3).

UNFORGIVENESS

Many believers do not receive answers to their prayers because somewhere along the line they have wronged someone, or they have been wronged by someone and have failed to humble themselves and seek reconciliation. In the Sermon on the Mount, Jesus said, *Therefore, if you are presenting your offering at the altar, and there remember that your brother has something against you, leave your offering there before the altar and go; first be reconciled to your brother, and then come and present your offering* (Matthew 5:23-24).

Unforgiveness in your heart creates a division in your relationship with God. Jesus states: *For if you forgive others for their transgressions, your heavenly Father will also forgive you. But if you do not forgive others, then your Father will not forgive your transgressions* (Matthew 6:14-15).

UNBELIEF

Doubt, fear, and worry are forms of unbelief. When present, they prevent faith from rising up within and will keep your prayers from being answered: *But he must ask in faith without any doubting, for the one who doubts is like the surf of the sea, driven and tossed by the wind. For that man ought not to expect that he will receive anything from the Lord* (James 1:6-7). Faith is the opposite of unbelief and is required by God in order for Him to respond: . . . *without faith it is impossible to please Him, for he who comes to God must believe that He is and that He is a rewarder of those who* [diligently] *seek Him* (Hebrews 11:6).

SELF-EXAMINATION

When the Apostle Paul wrote to the Corinthians, he pointed out that many of them were weak, sick, and had died because they had not judged (examined) themselves correctly. Many of these believers were *not* getting healed of their sickness and disease. They were praying yet remained sick. God definitely wants to answer all prayers, but He is bound by His Word, *For there is no partiality with God* (Romans 2:11). If we lack understanding of God's Word with respect to His wonderful promises, we can clearly miss out on many aspects of living an abundant life, such as freedom from disease and receiving a miraculous healing if we do become sick. God points this out Himself: *My people perish for lack of knowledge . . .* (Hosea 4:6). Therefore, learning from God's Word is imperative.

In Joshua 1:7 we are instructed to *Only be strong and very courageous; be careful to do according to all the law which Moses my servant commanded you; do not turn from it to the right or to the left, so that you may have success wherever you go.* By spending time in God's Word, we get to know His Word, and through this knowledge of God's Word, our . . . *senses* [get] *trained to discern good and evil* (Hebrews 5:14). As a result, we are capable of examining our lives and making corrections along the way: *But if we judged ourselves rightly, we would not be judged* (1 Corinthians 11:31).

HUMILITY

In humility, ask the Holy Spirit to reveal anything in your life that is not pleasing to God. Whatever He shows you ask for forgiveness, turn from it (repent), and thank the Lord for His forgiveness. When your heart is pure before God, it becomes easier to approach the throne of grace with boldness and to receive help from the Lord: *Therefore let us draw near with confidence to the throne of grace, so that we may receive mercy and find grace in time of need* (Hebrews 4:16). If your heart is heavy and does not feel pure, the Lord invites you to humbly seek Him for help. Those who humble themselves before God are rewarded: *Humble yourself in the presence of the Lord, and he will exalt you* (James 4:10); *for everyone who exalts himself will be humbled, and he who humbles himself will be exalted* (Luke 14:11).

KINDNESS

Your choice of kind words can bring forth healing to your body and balance to your soul: *Pleasant words are a honeycomb, sweet to the soul and healing to the bones* (Proverbs 16:24).

WORSHIP AND HONOR

Worshipping and honoring God for who He is brings with it many blessings, including healing: *But you shall serve the Lord your God, and He will bless your bread and your water; and I will remove sickness from your midst... I will fulfill the number of your days* (Exodus 23:25-26).

LOVE FOR GOD

Having a loving relationship with God will protect you and deliver you from disease. A powerful passage that supports this idea is Psalm 91:7-16: *A thousand may fall at your side, and ten thousand at your right hand, but it shall not approach you . . . For you have made the Lord, my refuge, even the Most High, your dwelling place. No evil will befall you, nor will any plague come near your tent . . . 'Because he has loved Me', says the Lord, 'therefore I will deliver him; I will set him securely on high, because he has known My name. He will call upon Me, and I will answer him; I will be with him in trouble, I will rescue him and honor him. With a long life will I satisfy him and let him see My salvation.'*

THE LORD PROMISES HEALING

The Lord heals. He promises over and over again that He will do this for you: *Bless the Lord, O my soul, and forget none of His benefits; who pardons all your iniquities, who heals all your diseases; who redeems your life from the pit, who crowns you with loving kindness and compassion* (Psalm 103:2-4); *Then they cried to the Lord in their trouble, and He saved them from their distresses. He sent His Word and healed them, He delivered them from their destructions* (Psalm 107:19-20); *O Lord my God, I cried to You for help, and You healed me* (Psalm 30:2).

Pay Attention

Knowing and clinging to God's Word is not only powerful, it is life itself: *My son, give attention to My words; incline your ear to My sayings . . . Do not let them depart from your sight; keep them in the midst of your heart. For they are life to those who find them and health to all their body* (Proverbs 4:20-22).

Speak God's Promises in Faith

The Word of God is living and active and sharper than any two-edged sword. When spoken in faith, it never returns empty but accomplishes the very thing God intends it to accomplish! God's Word—the Bible—is filled with promises that when acted upon in faith will accomplish much, even the miraculous. As believers, we can exercise our faith to command sickness to depart. Jesus granted us this authority (see Mark 16:17-18). He even said in John 14:12 that we will do greater works than He did, and that nothing would be impossible for us (see Matthew 17:20).

Speaking out God's Word is a means of calling in things that God has already given us by promise but has yet to physically manifest. When you speak out God's Word—His promises—you are tapping into the power of what God has already declared to be true concerning healing. When you speak out His promises you allow them to be set in motion to bring about miraculous results and healing.

It is Finished!

Our healing is a done deal! It has already been provided by Christ's sacrifice and God's promise to fulfill. If our hearts are right before God and we believe in what God has already said in His Word, we tap into the healing power that is available to us through the finished work on the cross: *But He was pierced through for our transgressions, He was crushed for our iniquities; the chastening for our well-being fell upon Him, and by His scourging we are healed* (Isaiah 53:5). We *are* healed! The Word does not say we *will be* or *may be* healed. It is a finished work.

Believing in a spiritual promise from God's Word will bring forth physical healing, providing prayer is not hindered and one does not give up. While this notion may challenge some, my personal testimony is a true story that supports this belief; and one that resulted in a miraculous healing. Scripture calls us to become *imitators of those who through faith and patience inherit the promises* (Hebrews 6:12). Therefore, imitate me. Imitate Daniel as he prayed, fasted, and persevered, until he inherited the promises (see Daniel 10)! God promises to perform on His Word: . . . *I am watching over My word to perform it* (Jeremiah 1:12). When we persistently believe in what God has said in His Word and expect it to happen personally for us, He will make it a reality in our lives. Your circumstances have no power over God's promises!

MOVE YOUR MOUNTAIN

Jesus said, *Have faith in God. Truly I say to you, whoever says to this mountain* [of sickness or whatever], '*Be taken up and cast into the sea,' and does not doubt in his heart, but believes that what he says is going to happen, it will be granted him. Therefore I say to you, all things for which you pray and ask, believe that you have received them, and they will be granted you* (Mark 11:22-24).

This same miracle-working faith is available to all: *This is the confidence which we have before Him, that, if we ask anything according to His will, He hears us. And if we know that He hears us in whatever we ask, we know that we have the requests which we have asked from Him* (1 John 5:14-15). Remember: . . . *faith comes from hearing, and hearing by the word of Christ* (Romans 10:17). The more of the Word that you have in your heart, the stronger your faith will become. And the stronger your faith, the more miracles you will experience. Take the time and study the written Word of the One who created you. He loves you and is... *able to do far more abundantly beyond all you ask or think...* (Ephesians 3:20).

God's Endorsement

Jesus is the same yesterday, today, and forever. He is our Great Physician and can heal in a variety of ways, providing they are in accordance with what He has already declared in His Word—our job is simply to believe and act on His promises.

In June 2002, while on a listing appointment with a couple who were planning a move, the wife, Rebecca, became intrigued with the healing miracle that happened in my life. On two occasions, during the time it took me to list and sell her home, Rebecca and I spoke intently about what I went through and the supporting Bible verses that I followed during the period of the illness. In December of that same year, Rebecca shared the following incredible story with me:

Amy is a friend of mine who I have known since childhood. She had been fighting liver and pancreatic cancer for a while. Back in August, the doctors stopped her treatment, and she was sent to hospice care. She was given two weeks to live. At that time, the Lord spoke to me audibly. The Lord said to me, "Rebecca, I want you to go to Amy and teach her what you learned about healing while you were in Minnesota and give her Jeff's CD."

Rebecca continued, telling me that she had never experienced anything like this. She informed me she had never witnessed to her friend Amy about the Lord, but since she heard God's audible voice and since Amy had only days to live, she went on her assigned mission to speak to her.

Rebecca told me that Amy listened intently to what she shared with her and subsequently listened to the CD. Amy then asked for a Bible and for healing tapes. She read, and she listened. She asked for praise CDs. She wrote out sticky notes of Bible verses and affirmations of her expected healing and posted them on the walls. She spoke them aloud daily. She made changes to her diet. She duplicated all the activities that I had done while sick in 2001. Day by day, Amy gained strength, and after four months, she had no more cancer in her body! The doctors could not explain it—she is perfectly healthy now!

Beyond Belief? No. Not at all! I have experienced this same miraculous power by believing and acting on God's promises. And He has encouraged me to share what I have learned and to remind others that He loves them and is no respecter of persons. Therefore, I now encourage you to be *imitators of those who through faith and patience inherit the promises* (Hebrews 6:12).

. . . be imitators of those who through faith and patience inherit the promises

---

CHAPTER 7

— Salvation Prayer —

*Having a personal relationship with Jesus Christ, the Son of God,
is essential to receiving all the benefits God has to offer you—both
in this life and the life to come. For Jesus said, . . . I came that you
might have life, and have it abundantly.*
JOHN 10:10

CHAPTER 7

According to 1 Timothy 2:5, *There is one God, and one Mediator also between God and men, the man Christ Jesus.* Jesus is our bridge to God; the only way to heaven. Jesus said, *I am the Way, the Truth and the Life; no one comes to the Father except through Me.*

For anyone to see God and get into heaven they must first receive Jesus into their heart in a personal way. For . . . *there is salvation in no one else; for there is no other name under heaven that has been given to men by which we must be saved* (Acts 4:12). Jesus is that name: . . . *God has given us eternal life, and this life is in His Son. He who has the Son has the life; he who does not have the Son of God does not have the life* (1 John 5:11-12).

If you have never invited Jesus into your heart, or if you are not sure about your relationship with Him, I invite you to pray this prayer from your heart; it will change your life for good, as well as change your life forever:

Heavenly Father,

I come to You in all honesty asking for Your help.

I know that I have messed up;

I've done things I'm not proud of and have sinned

against You and against others.

I have lived selfishly, for myself.

Please, forgive me of all this.

I want to change and ask for Your help to do so.

I believe that Jesus died on the cross for my sins.

I also believe that

He rose again from the dead and lives forever.

Lord Jesus, I need You.

I want to turn away from my sins.

I ask for Your help. Come into my heart and

give me strength to live for You.

Thank You for forgiving me, saving me, and giving me

eternal life.

Help me to become the person You want me to be.

Thank You.

In Jesus' name,

Amen

CHAPTER 8

— TWENTY-EIGHT VERSES FROM THE HOSPITAL —

CHAPTER 8

The following twenty-eight verses are the particular Bible verses that the Lord put on my heart while I spent those twenty-eight days in the hospital. These verses gave me strength and ministered to my visitors and the hospital staff as well.

DAY 1

James 1:2-4, has always given me strength—before, during and after my hospital stay: *Consider it all joy my brethren, when you encounter various trials, knowing that the testing of your faith produces endurance. And let endurance have its perfect result, that you may be perfect and complete, lacking in nothing.*

DAY 2

I stood on this promise all the way through my journey, knowing that I would be restored in the end: *Therefore humble yourselves under the mighty hand of God, that He may exalt you at the proper time, casting all your anxiety (cares) upon Him, because He cares for you. Be of sober spirit, be on the alert. Your adversary, the devil, prowls about like a roaring lion, seeking someone to devour. But resist him, firm in your faith, knowing that the same experiences of suffering are being accomplished by your brethren who are in the world. And after you have suffered for a little while, the God of all grace, who called you to His eternal glory in Christ, shall Himself, restore, strengthen, perfect, establish and confirm you* (1 Peter 5:6-10).

DAY 3

The third day in the hospital was the day they performed the bone marrow biopsy; I cannot think of a more fitting verse: *For the*

Word of God is living and active and sharper than any two-edged sword, and piercing as far as the division of soul and spirit, of both joints and marrow, and able to judge the thoughts and intentions of the heart (Hebrews 4:12).

DAY 4

No weapon or sickness from the enemy will prosper or be victorious over me! If God said it then it's settled: *No weapon that is formed against you will prosper . . .*(Isaiah 54:17).

DAY 5

The powerful promises of Psalm 34:7, 17, and 19 seemed fitting because our Prayer/Care Pastor had seen the angel Gabriel standing outside my hospital room door: *The angel of the Lord encamps around those who fear Him, and rescues them . . . The righteous cry, and the Lord hears and delivers them out of all their troubles . . . Many are the afflictions of the righteous, but the Lord delivers him out of them all.*

DAY 6

At no time did I believe my life would end as a result of this ordeal. Although the doctors, the textbooks, and all those Internet articles indicated the odds were greatly against me, I knew that if God was for me, then nothing could be against me: *For I know the plans that I have for you, declares the Lord, plans for welfare and not for calamity, to give you a future and a hope* (Jeremiah 29:11).

DAY 7

I received this as a personal promise and by having the Word of God in my heart, it resulted in health to my entire body: *My son, give attention to My words; incline your ear to My sayings. Do not let them depart from your sight; keep them in the midst of your heart. For they are life to those who find them and health to their whole body* (Proverbs 4:20-22).

DAY 8

Throughout this strange and challenging time, I kept rejoicing, knowing that, at the revelation of His glory (my perfect health report), I would rejoice with exultation: *Beloved, do not be surprised at the fiery ordeal among you, which comes upon you for your testing, as though some strange thing were happening to you; but to the degree that you share the sufferings of Christ, keep on rejoicing; so that also at the revelation of His glory, you may rejoice with exultation* (1 Peter 4:12-13).

DAY 9

If we abide in Christ, He will give us all things for which we ask. If we ask anything according to His will, He will give it to us, and the outcome is our being filled with joy: *If you abide in Me, and My words abide in you, ask whatever you wish, and it shall be done for you. My Father is glorified by this, that you bear much fruit, and so prove to be My disciples. Just as the Father has loved Me, I have also loved you. Abide in My love. If you keep My commandments, you will abide in My love; just as I have kept My Father's commandments, and abide in His love. These things I have spoken to you, that My joy may be in you, and that your joy may be made full* (John 15:7-11).

DAY 10

If we abide in Him (do the things that are pleasing in His sight), then whatever we ask we will receive from Him: *And whatever we ask we receive from Him, because we keep His commandments and do the things that are pleasing in His sight* (1 John 3:22).

DAY 11

No passage of scripture indicates *when* we will receive an answer to our prayer but that we *have* received it when we ask! We are to have confidence in this! This is why it is critical, when we pray according to God's will, that we trust Him to deliver the answer in *His perfect timing*. Most often it is the waiting that tests our faith. God is rarely early, but He is never late! Wait on the Lord. Trust Him, and He will fulfill His promises: *This is the confidence which we have before Him, that, if we ask anything according to His will, He hears us. And if we know that He hears us in whatever we ask, we know that we have the requests which we have asked from Him* (1 John 5:14-15).

DAY 12

According to 2 Timothy 1:7, God empowers believers so that they will not be overcome by fear; He gives us a spirit of love, power, and a sound mind: *For God has not given us a spirit of fear, but of love, power and a sound mind.*

DAY 13

If you are facing a challenge in your life, pray, expect, stand firm in your faith, do not shrink back, and know that there is a great reward if you don't throw away your trust and confidence in what the Lord has promised: *And we desire that each one of you show the same diligence so as to realize the full assurance of hope until the end, so that you may not be sluggish, but imitators of those who through faith and patience inherit the promises . . . Therefore, do not throw away your confidence, which has a great reward. For you have need of endurance, so that when you have done the will of God, you may receive what was promised . . . But My righteous one shall live by faith; and if he shrinks back, My soul has no pleasure in him* (Hebrews 6:11-12; 10:35-38).

Day 14

Each day I expected my blood numbers to miraculously return to normal, but they never did while in the hospital. But I did not get discouraged. I repeatedly told myself to focus not on what I could see but on what I could not see—not to focus on the circumstance but on the promise: *For we walk by faith, not by sight* (2 Corinthians 5:7).

Day 15

Proverbs 3:5-8 says, *Trust in the Lord with all your heart, and do not lean on your own understanding. In all your ways acknowledge Him, and He will make your paths straight. Do not be wise in your own eyes; fear the Lord and turn away from evil. It will be healing to your body and marrow to your bones.* I often catch myself not following the first part of this passage, as I am quite the thinker. All too often I try to figure things out in my *mind* instead of trusting the Lord with all my *heart*. Note the powerful result that being humble, revering God, and turning from evil has; it brings healing to the body and marrow to the bones!

Day 16

As a husband, I am to honor my wife, just as Christ honors the church. Christ gave Himself up for the church, and, as a husband, I am to do the same. But it does not end there. Husbands are to love their wives as they would love their own bodies, nourishing and cherishing them just as Christ does the church: *Husbands, love your wives, just as Christ also loved the Church and gave Himself up for her, so that He might sanctify her, having cleansed her by the washing of water with the Word, that He might present to Himself the church in all her glory, having no spot or wrinkle or any such thing; but that she would be holy and blameless. So husbands ought also to love their own wives as their own bodies ... each individual among you also is to love his own wife even as himself, and the wife must see to it that she respects her husband* (Ephesians 5:25–28, 33).

DAY 17

This prayer became the framework for one of the best-selling books in the U.S. in 2001: *Now Jabez called on the God of Israel, saying, 'Oh that You would bless me indeed, and enlarge my border, and that Thy hand might be with me, and that You would keep me from harm, that it may not pain me!'* (1 Chronicles 4:10). Jabez set an example for me, as I boldly petitioned God: bless me indeed with a blessing so certain that all are amazed; enlarge my border by giving me greater responsibility and opportunity for You; may Your hand be with me to guide me through every twist and turn I encounter; and keep me from harm and from the snares of the devil so that it may not pain me. Scripture says God granted Jabez his request. He granted mine as well!

DAY 18

This powerful verse clearly indicates that our healing is a finished work; Jesus paid the price for our sins and our diseases on the cross: *And He Himself bore our sins in His body on the cross, so that we might die to sin and live to righteousness; for by His wounds [stripes] you were healed* (1 Peter 2:24).

DAY 19

This verse came to me and reinforced my responsibility of honoring my wife; if we fail to do so our prayers may be hindered: *You husbands in the same way, live with your wives in an understanding way, as with someone weaker, since she is a woman; and show her honor as a fellow heir of the grace of life, so that your prayers may not be hindered* (1 Peter 3:7).

DAY 20

Jesus says that He came to destroy the works of the devil—to give life and to give it abundantly! This is the good news that is available to all who believe: *The thief comes only to steal and kill and destroy; I came that they may have life, and have it abundantly* (John 10:10).

DAY 21

Patience and trust is key to *waiting on the Lord.* I will admit that it is not always easy to do, but the reward is the receiving of God's promise. He is faithful to always keep His Word. His timing is perfect—better than anything we could ever plan out on our own. This passage has a special meaning to me due to my experience; I was in need of physical strength since any attempt to run (or walk at length) would cause me to tire and grow weary. But God promised that if I trusted Him and waited on Him I would gain new strength: *Yet those who wait for the Lord will gain new strength; they will mount up with wings like eagles; they will run and not get tired; they will walk and not become weary* (Isaiah 40:31).

DAY 22

Regarding others as more important than ourselves is virtually impossible to do on our own. In other words, without the love of God flowing though us, it would be very unlikely for us to truly feel this way toward anyone else. We may want to live this way and act this way toward others, but only when we allow God's perfect love to flow through us, can we truly put the interests of others ahead of our own: *Do nothing from selfishness or empty conceit, but with humility of mind regard one another as more important than yourselves; do not merely look out for your own personal interests, but also for the interests of others* (Philippians 2:3-4).

DAY 23

This passage is so awesome; God is able to do things for us that exceed our capacity to ask or even imagine—providing we are asking in faith—for faith is the power that works within us: *Now to him who is able to do far more abundantly beyond all that we ask or think, according to the power that works within us . . . to Him be the glory* (Ephesians 3:20-21).

DAY 24

This verse seemed fitting as it deals with the bones. As the Lord put this on my heart, I was crying for the Lord's gracious mercy to rescue me with healing: *Be gracious to me, O Lord, for I am pining away; heal me, O Lord, for my bones are dismayed* (Psalm 6:2).

DAY 25

Jeremiah 30:17 is short, sweet, and direct; I received this verse as a promise from the Lord: *For I will restore you to health and I will heal you of your wounds, declares the Lord . . .*

DAY 26

Of the many wonderful things God does out of His unconditional loving kindness and compassion, He heals ALL of our diseases; He satisfies our lives with good things so we gain strength—even to the degree of looking and feeling younger: *Bless the Lord, O my soul, and forget none of His benefits, who pardons all your iniquities, who heals all your diseases; who redeems your life from the pit, who crowns you with loving kindness and compassion; who satisfies your years with good things, so that your youth is renewed like the eagle* (Psalm 103:2-5).

Day 27

According to 1 John 5:4, *For whatever is born of God overcomes the world; and this is the victory that has overcome the world—our faith.* I love this verse. It speaks of the power within us, given by God and through our faith, to overcome anything that Satan can dish out. As one who has accepted Christ as Savior and Lord (born again), I already have the victory through faith!

Day 28

This passage was given to me as a word from the Lord by a pastor from Nigeria with whom I crossed paths as I was checking out of the hospital. This verse was initially spoken by Jesus when He was told to come and heal Lazarus after hearing he was sick: *. . . this sickness is not to end in death, but for the glory of God, so that the Son of God may be glorified by it* (John 11:4).

ABOUT THE AUTHOR

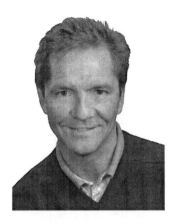

In 2001, successful real estate broker Jeff Scislow began what would be his toughest battle; the battle for his life. Diagnosed with aplastic anemia, he was told that his prognosis was grim and to get his affairs in order. Through prayer, faithful expectation and sheer determination, Jeff optimistically ran that race and today, he is in perfect health.

After his miraculous recovery he continued to build upon his successful real estate business while penning two books - *The Promise*, which is now available in multiple languages, and *Journey to a Miracle.*

Jeff resides in Apple Valley, Minnesota. He regularly speaks on a variety of business and inspirational topics around the world.

ACKNOWLEDGMENTS

We all experience challenges in life, and it is during those difficult times that we need others the most. I wish to sincerely thank every person that prayed and showed concern for me during my darkest hour.

To my wife Susy: You not only supported me emotionally and through prayer but managed the office, our household, and our four children. On top of this, you went on listing appointments in my absence in order to keep the business rolling. You were incredible. Thank you from the bottom of my heart.

To my children: Although you were all quite young at the time, I commend you for being strong in your faith, knowing and believing that your dad would come home again and that he would live and not die.

To my parents, my brothers, my sister, and my entire family: I thank you for being there for me and believing this was just another challenge for Jeff—one that he'd overcome. I can assure you, I would never want to have faced it without Jesus. This I know: I *can* do all things through Christ who strengthens me.

To my doctors and my nurses: I really wish to thank you for being there on a daily basis for me. Taking care of sick people really takes a special talent and a special heart. You are all incredibly patient, very understanding, and empathetic. You are *givers*, and each of you was more than that. In many ways, I may not have been your *normal* patient. I chose to be joyful in order to combat sorrow and chose faith to overcome fear. In the end, the Lord healed me and granted me victory over a killer disease. I am glad you had the opportunity to witness it first-hand.

To my special friends who played a direct role in my journey, Pastor Dave Housholder, Shirley, Pastor Holmes, Paul, Pastor Moe, Regan, Doug Stanton, Monique, Marjorie Cole, Elaine Bonn, and John Kittleson: Thank you so much for hearing the Word of the Lord as He spoke to you and used you to play a part in my miracle. I will always pray blessings over you.

To all who prayed for me and took time to encourage me during this time: Your visits, calls, letters, cards, and emails meant more than you can imagine. They inspired me to *fight the good fight*. Yes, God said He would show Himself strong through me before the eyes of many people, but He used each of you to play a part. You've experienced first-hand the power your encouragement had upon me. Thank you. Now, continue to do the same in the lives of others.

Expressions of kindness and gratitude can move mountains, melt hearts, and heal wounds.

– JEFF SCISLOW

RECOMMENDED RESOURCES

BOOKS, WEBSITES, AND MINISTRIES

There were many valuable resources that I encountered on my *Journey to a Miracle*. I read books, and visited countless websites. I also met a number of individuals and tried their products and got to know their ministries. Those listed below have been the greatest blessing to me.

BOOKS

HEALING PRAYER
BY REGINALD CHERRY, M.D.

This book discusses God's divine intervention in medicine, faith, and prayer. The author is right on when it comes to healing and prayer. I have found his material scripturally accurate and educational to me.

www.DrCherry.org

LIVE RIGHT 4 YOUR TYPE
BY DR. PETER D'ADAMO

An excellent book that explores an individualized prescription for maximizing health, metabolism, and vitality in every stage of life, based on a person's blood type. In 1999, *Eat Right 4 Your Type*,

Dr. D'Adamo's earlier book on this topic, was named one of the ten most influential health books ever written.

www.dadamo.com

A MORE EXCELLENT WAY
BY PASTOR HENRY WRIGHT

A deep teaching on the spiritual roots of disease. Pastor Wright explores a variety of human emotions and life experiences that birth specific diseases within the body and offers sound Biblical advice on how to bring forth healing.

www.pleasantvalleychurch.net

GOD'S CREATIVE POWER FOR HEALING
BY CHARLES CAPPS

This is a wonderful, forty-six page book, which has sold more than 4 million copies! In it, you will learn how you can release the ability of God to heal by the words from your own mouth!

www.charlescapps.com

WEBSITES
WWW.DRDAY.COM

Dr. Lorraine Day is an internationally acclaimed orthopedic trauma surgeon and bestselling author. Dr. Day was diagnosed with invasive breast cancer but rejected standard therapies because of their destructive side effects that often lead to death. She chose instead to rebuild her immune system using the natural, simple, inexpensive therapies designed by God and outlined in the Bible so her body could heal itself.

www.HerbDoc.com

According to the website of Dr. Richard Schulze, you will *learn how to take responsibility for your own health! The purpose of this website is to inspire you to take responsibility for your own health and to cure yourself. All diseases are curable, but not all the people! It is all up to you. It is your choice whether you are going to be curable or not.*

Ministries

Healing Center International (Elaine Bonn)

This is a wonderful place to go to have intelligent, well-trained Christian counselors listen to you, answer your questions, and then pray specifically for your needs. There is a genuine desire to get to the root of any issue or problem and to come against it in Jesus' name, expecting the Lord to move and heal (whether physical, emotional, spiritual, financial, or whatever).

www.healingcenterintl.org

Life Recovery (Marjorie Cole)

Author of *Taking the Devil to Court*, Marjorie Cole is an expert on generational curses and praying for deliverance. Her prayer and counseling sessions are helpful in understanding the potential cause of diseases. Additionally, she maintains a wealth of knowledge with respect to spiritual warfare and clearly understands that *our struggle is not against flesh and blood . . . but against the spiritual forces of wickedness in the heavenly places* (Ephesians 6:12).

www.LifeRecovery.com

a Book's Mind

Whether you want to purchase bulk copies of
Journey to a Miracle
or buy another book for a friend, get it now at:
www.JourneyToAMiracle.com

If you have a book that you would like to publish,
contact A Book's Mind: info@abooksmind.com.

www.abooksmind.com

CPSIA information can be obtained at www.ICGtesting.com
Printed in the USA
BVOW02s0031120314

347349BV00008B/145/P